The Image of Professional Nursing
Strategies for Action

DATE DUE

The Image of Professional Nursing

Strategies for Action

LEANN STRASEN, RN, MBA, DPA
Corporate Senior Vice President
Hospital Group
National Medical Enterprises, Inc.
Santa Monica, California

J. B. Lippincott Company
Philadelphia
New York   London   Hagerstown

Sponsoring Editor: Donna L. Hilton, RN, BSN
Production Manager: Janet Greenwood
Production: Publishers' WorkGroup
Compositor: Bucks County Type & Design
Printer/Binder: R. R. Donnelley & Sons Company

6 5 4 3 2 1

Library of Congress Cataloging-in-Publication Data
Strasen, Leann.
   The image of professional nursing: strategies for action/Leann
Strasen.
      p. cm.
   Includes bibliographical references and index.
   ISBN 0–397–54815–X
   1. Nurses—Psychology.   2. Self-perception.   I. Title
   [DNLM: 1. Achievement.   2. Nurses—psychology.   3. Professional
Practice.   4. Self Concept.   5. Social Perception.   WY 87 S895i]
RT86.S74   1992
610.73'019—dc20
DNLM/DLC
for Library of Congress   91–14166
                                                                       CIP

This book is dedicated to professional nurses who are frustrated, disenchanted, or unhappy with their personal or professional lives. The bad news is that you are responsible for your situation; the good news is that you are responsible for your future happiness and success. You can take immediate action to improve your personal and professional life. JUST DO IT!

There are a number of people I'd like to acknowledge who have significantly influenced the writing of this book: Helene Mierendorf, who socialized me to believe I could do anything I set my mind to; Edwin Mierendorf, who always gave me a B+ when I was striving for an A+; Shaggy Strasen, our 17-year-old cock-a-poo who acts like a puppy because we treat him like a puppy and have never told him how old he really is; Peter Strasen, who encourages me to keep putting pictures of my goals up on the refrigerator, no matter how off-the-wall they are; and my colleagues, who reinforce my ideas by sharing their successes with me. I would especially like to thank Donna Hilton, my editor, for taking the risk and supporting this nontraditional effort to enhance the image of the nursing profession. Donna allowed me to say the things I felt needed to be said, even those that no one enjoys hearing. Without her support, this project would not have become a reality.

Preface

The image of nursing is an issue that has concerned the profession for decades. The only current topic that seems to be talked about more is the nursing shortage. The issue has been discussed and reviewed, and volumes of recommendations have been written by study committees, professional organizations, and presidential advisory committees. However, nothing seems to change.

Perhaps changes do not occur because the recommendations focus primarily on actions that groups outside of nursing might take to improve the image of nursing. These recommendations include suggestions that

1. The media needs to portray nursing in a more positive light.
2. Physicians need to treat nurses better and hospitals need to develop formal programs designed to improve physician–nurse relationships (CAHHS, 1989).
3. Hospitals need to evaluate and improve nurse salary and compensation packages.
4. Hospital organizations, in conjunction with nursing professional organizations, should initiate statewide professional image recruitment campaigns (CAHHS, 1989).

Each of these recommendations depends on a group outside the profession of nursing taking action or making changes. When these groups do not take such action, the problems remain unchanged.

However, if we in the profession develop recommendations that focus on nurses themselves taking action toward change, we most likely would have a better chance of improving the image of nursing.

In other situations, most people have learned that they really cannot change or control anyone but themselves. Having realized this, they deal with the world on those terms and become less frustrated. This seems to accomplish more because the focus of the person's energy is on their own actions rather than on the actions of others.

Following that logic, this book is based on the hypothesis that effective and lasting changes for the image of professional nursing must focus on changing the self-image of each individual nurse. As a result, the self-image model has been used as the conceptual framework for the book because it forces us to focus our efforts on ourselves.

According to the self-image model, a person's thoughts and beliefs determine that person's self-image. Self-image determines actions, performance, and achievements. Each nurse's actions and achievements, in turn, affect the collective image of professional nursing. The image of professional nursing then supports or alters the individual nurse's self-image. Figure A-1 outlines these relationships.

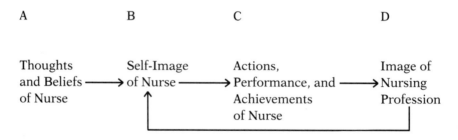

Figure A-1. Self-Image Model for the Nursing Profession

Most of the efforts to improve the image of nursing have been aimed at point *D* in the model, that is, on the already established professional image of nursing. This focus does not appear to have been effective, and little change has been evident because it is difficult to develop a concrete, effective plan of action to change the image of such a large group of people.

This book, on the other hand, focuses on point *A* in the model. Changing the thoughts and beliefs of individual nurses will in turn determine their self-image and subsequently their actions and performance. If enough nurses can enhance their self-images, the image and achievements of the entire profession can improve. This approach seems to be a more realistic way of tackling the problem.

Using contemporary literature on the psychology of women and on gender socialization, this book offers explanations about why the image of nursing is where it is in the early 1990s. It also uses the self-image model to offer suggestions to nurses on how to improve the image of nursing in the 1990s and beyond. Attainment of this goal is not easy. The concept and plan of action is, however, simple. The acid test lies in whether a majority of nurses desire to improve the quality of their personal and professional lives by improving their own self-images.

Other articles and books on this topic have stressed the impact of gender socialization, sexism, and stereotyping on the profession of nursing and the performance and achievements of nurses (Muff, 1982). This book outlines the strong impact, influence, and effect that gender socialization has on female nurses; however, the emphasis is on proactive ways to respond to these issues.

I do not discuss the challenge to change gender and nurse socialization in this book. I leave that work to others. It seems that even if strong efforts to change or alter traditional gender socialization are accomplished, people must still live in the real world and face varying and challenging situations with physical, social, and emotional factors that may compromise their lives or are perceived as being "unfair." Even if we eliminate all forms of sex discrimination or stereotyping, people will have to deal with the effects of broken families, socioeconomic factors, physical illnesses, trauma, losses, failures, etc. Therefore, people will still have to learn to respond positively to adverse situations.

The first chapter in this book acknowledges the unique factors that have contributed to the current position of female nurses and the profession of nursing. The second chapter describes three self-image models that explain how self-image drives our actions, behaviors, and achievements. The remainder of the book then focuses on how individual nurses can take responsibility for their lives from this point on to be successful, rather than blaming society, the world, physicians, fellow nurses, parents, the government, hospital administrators, etc. It seems that in the past, placing the blame on others has not helped anyone to move ahead, or to take action to better themselves. The bulk of the book outlines strategies that novice and experienced clinical nurses, nurse managers, and nurse executives can implement to enhance their self-images and performance. Chapter Seven closes with proposed strategies for nurses in formal groups and organizations to enhance the image of the profession after they have enhanced their own self-image and self-esteem.

Leann Strasen, RN, MBA, DPA

Contents

The Image of Professional Nursing
Strategies for Action

1

Gender Socialization and the Image of Professional Nursing

The image of the nursing profession has been a popular topic of discussion in the past decade, but this discussion seems to have resulted in few actions that have had any positive impact on the overall image of the profession. In contrast, however, a number of trends in nurses' professional thinking and behavior appear to have had an effect on the image of the profession. Contemporary writing in the fields of psychology and sociology focusing on women's issues offer empirical data to support these observations. Although the purpose of reviewing this literature was to focus not on women's issues but on professional nursing issues, it became very apparent during my research that the image of professional nursing could not be responsibly discussed without acknowledging the relevance of contemporary literature in these areas.

Over the past two decades, much has been written about the impact of gender socialization on men and women. The literature supports the observation that many of the behavioral trends in nursing are actually women's issues that are "professionalized" because of the high percentage of women in the profession of nursing. This chapter outlines the components of gender socialization and the specific issues this socialization raises for women and nurses.

Female nurses are the largest single group of professionals in the health care industry. Although increasing numbers of men are entering the nursing profession, more than 96% of nurses are women. Although the intent of this book is not to ignore the impact of men on the

KEY CHAPTER CONCEPTS

Key Concept #1

Self-image, or self-concept, is the set of beliefs and images we hold true about ourselves based on our specific socialization.

Key Concept #2

The development of gender self-concept begins at the age of two and has significant implications for the roles, responsibilities, and capabilities of the individual.

Key Concept #3

The traditional gender socialization of women has fostered dependence, a strong commitment to relationships with others, an external locus of control, and a self-concept that can be very self-limiting.

Key Concept #4

The traditional gender socialization of men has fostered independence, reliance on self or an internal locus of control, and high self-esteem.

Key Concept #5

Self-esteem measures how much you like and approve of your self-image.

profession, this chapter describes the impact of gender socialization on women in general and on the profession of nursing.

Despite the focus on female nurses, this book provides insights into the thoughts and actions of nurses that can assist male nurses, managers, and administrators to work more effectively with female nurses on a day-to-day basis.

CULTURE AND SOCIALIZATION

Culture is the set of definitions of reality held in common by a group of individuals who share a distinctive way of life (Kluckholn, 1962). Culture includes the pattern of expectations concerning the behaviors, beliefs, and actions of members of a particular group or society.

The culture of a society includes complex sets of gender norms or expectations concerning male and female behavior—that is, how they are to think, act, and perform within the society. In general, male and female behavioral traits are learned patterns of behavior rather than predetermined biological conditions. These gender norms are powerful mechanisms that control human behavior in subtle ways.

Gender role, or sex role, is the expectation of appropriate male and female behavior found in the attitudes and beliefs of a particular society. "Gender socialization" is the term used to describe the process by which these sex roles are learned by the individual (Anderson, 1983; Muff, 1982; Kalisch and Kalisch, 1982). The process of gender socialization acts as a powerful method to control the actions of men and women. Traditionally, Western sex role socialization has directed women to avoid power, achievement, and independence, while training men to avoid exhibiting emotional and nurturing behaviors (Tolson, 1977). According to **Key Concept #4**, gender is a sociological way of categorizing individuals based on their biological sex. Categorization is essential in a complex society because it helps individuals relate to different groups within that society. According to **Key Concept #2**, individuals learn at a very young age to identify relationships with others by categorizing them into broad categories such as male, female, mother, father, teacher, brother, etc. Without the use of such broad categories, children and adults would have significant difficulty relating to others in our society.

On the other hand, when such a method of categorization becomes more important than the characteristics of a particular individual, stereotyping occurs. Stereotyping is categorizing and interrelating with individuals solely on the basis of the expected traits of the role category rather than on the basis of the individual. For example, stereotyping becomes a problem when a woman, despite her exceptional educational and career accomplishments, is not even considered for a promotion because she is stereotyped as being a short-term female employee who will soon leave to have a child.

It is important for nurses to realize that the concept of stereotyping exists, to understand its potential influence, and to take steps to counteract and overcome its influence on their performance and achievements. It is useless to dwell on the unfairness of stereotyping. Instead, we should recognize that the social stereotyping of men, women, or nurses cannot be completely changed in the short term. However, the influence of stereotyping on individuals can be overcome, and over time the stereotyping of women in general and female nurses can also change.

THE DEVELOPMENT OF
SELF-CONCEPT

Key Concept #1 articulates that self-concept and self-image are two terms that can be used interchangeably to describe the set of beliefs and images you hold true about yourself. According to *Key Concept #5*, self-esteem, self-respect, and self-worth are three terms that measure how much you like and approve of your self-concept or self-image.

Ideal self-image, on the other hand, is the picture of the person you believe you should be. When an individual's self-image and ideal self-image are drastically different, that person will have a low level of self-esteem. An individual whose self-image and ideal self are similar will have a high level of self-esteem.

People are not born with the beliefs and images that determine their self-image. Children learn self-image by interacting with their environment, family, and reference groups. Rosenberg (1979) reported that individuals' beliefs about their talents and abilities are strongly influenced by the people around them. Social psychologist George Herbert Mead (1934) argued that the development of self-concept is a cognitive process learned by children when playing the role of their same-sex significant other. Mead focused on the importance of play as a very significant part of gender socialization that teaches children how to relate to their environment.

Sanford and Donovan (1984) wrote that "being born into a particular family is like walking in on a party that has been going on for some time." The newborn child is in some ways similar to an intruder joining an already established group. The birth of a child abruptly alters all established family relationships, and the way in which family members react to the new child has a significant impact on that child's self-image. Specific family factors that affect a child's early self-image include the quality of the parents' relationship with each other, the child's birth order, the socioeconomic status of the family, pre-existing family conditions such as illness, the size of the family, the self-esteem of each parent, the difficulty of the mother's labor and delivery, and the gender of the child.

Erikson (1980) studied individual life cycles and the development of identity in the child. His research identified a number of stages that individuals pass through in their growth and development. His first four stages are (1) trust versus mistrust, which is experienced at one year of age; (2) autonomy versus shame and doubt, which is experienced at two to three years of age; (3) initiative versus guilt, which is experienced at four to five years of age; and (4) industry versus inferiority, which is experienced when the child enters school. Sex role socialization typically begins between the ages of four and five.

In the industry versus inferiority stage, the child spends most of the time playing. This play helps a child to master experiences for future growth and development by experimenting and sharing with other children. The child learns to win recognition by producing things that develop the child's sense of industry and experiences pleasure and recognition by completing tasks. On the other hand, if play does not stimulate industry in a child, a sense of inferiority and inadequacy may result.

Development of
Gender Self-Concept

The earliest form of self-concept learned is that of being male or female. In learning gender self-concept, the individual learns an array of specific expectations, roles, and responsibilities that accompany this male or female self-concept. The gender socialization process defines the self, the external world and one's place in it, and others and their relationship to the individual.

The traditional differences between female and male socialization are discussed in this section using broad generalizations about the traditional and typical socialization trends. Although there are exceptions to these socialization trends for both males and females, this section will focus on the way a majority of males and females in our society have been socialized in gender roles.

Children learn how significant and accepted they are from their parents' touch, nonverbal communications, tone of voice, and the amount of attention they receive. This communication significantly affects the early development of the child's self-esteem. Studies have shown that historically parents preferred having boys to girls (Sanford and Donovan, 1984). Through verbal and nonverbal communication they experience from their parents, girls learn at a very young age that they are less significant than boys.

The most crucial period in the formation of gender identity seems to be from age three to six. In this period, boys tend to receive more negative reinforcement for gender-inappropriate behavior than girls do from parents. Boys also receive more pressure, praise, encouragement, and punishment to accomplish specific goals.

Traditional gender socialization has taught boys to be independent, active, and aggressive and girls to be dependent, verbal, and social. Girls traditionally have been taught to have low aspirations because historically there have been so few roles and opportunities for them other than those of wife and mother.

Rabban (1950) reported that at the age of three, children prefer to be more like their mothers. By age five, however, most boys and a significant minority of girls prefer to be like their fathers (Brown, 1956). Hartley (1959) studied the way in which young boys and girls perceive the difference between boys and girls and between adult men and women. His results showed that all children perceive that the male role has superior status and privilege in society.

Despite these socialization differences, evidence shows that from a psychological perspective there is actually greater variability within the genders than between genders (Maccoby & Jacklin, 1974). Specifically, there are greater psychological differences between girls and women and between boys and men than there are between boys and girls or women and men.

The mother–child relationship is believed to have an extremely powerful influence on children of both sexes. A mother's specific words have a strong impact on the development of her child's self-image. They are accepted and internalized by the child whether or not they are true and whether or not they reflect inadequacies of the mother or the child. Criticisms or negative words from a mother have a great impact on children because they carry the threat of withholding parental love that is very important for a child.

TRADITIONAL SOCIALIZATION OF MEN AND WOMEN

The traditional socialization of women has been directed at preparing them to be good wives, mothers, and homemakers; men, on the other hand, have been socialized to become successful breadwinners. For women, careers outside the home have been acknowledged only as a way to spend time before marriage or after the children were grown. Furthermore, these careers have essentially been limited to helping or nurturing roles, such as being a secretary, nurse, teacher, or waitress.

Traditionally, women have been socialized to be people- and relationship-oriented. They have been taught to be helpful and pleasant, never to show anger, never to question authority figures, never to say no, never to bother others, never to be selfish or concerned about themselves, and to focus on making other people happy and comfortable. They have been taught to play nicely with others and never to compete or try to show off.

Men, on the other hand, have generally been socialized to be strong and to show this strength by proclaiming their accomplishments. They have been taught to speak up for themselves and never to cry. They have been taught that "nice guys finish last" and that they should aggressively "go for" whatever they want because they can count only on themselves.

Sociologists describe this sex role socialization as "instrumental" for men and "expressive" for women. The characteristics of instrumental socialization include the ability to compete, aggressiveness, and the ability to lead and to wield power to accomplish tasks. Expressive socialization includes learning to nurture, to be affiliative, and to be sensitive to the needs of others.

Elementary school texts have traditionally portrayed boys as the ones who make things happen and girls as those who watch things happen. Girls learn that external factors control their lives; boys learn that they are supposed to control external factors in order to determine their own success.

Rheingold and Cook (1975) observed that girls' toys tended to be less varied in type than boys' and that their play was largely limited to the home setting. Boys' toys, on the other hand, tended to have greater competency-eliciting potential and encouraged flexibility, diversity, and improvisation. Lever (1976) observed fifth-grade children in his research and noted that boys tended to play games that had goals and rules, while girls' games most often did not. Girls tended to play games that involved repetitious rituals such as jumping rope; boys' games were not repetitious and usually required and developed physical and mental skills. Lever concluded that boys' socialization assists them in acquiring the leadership and organizational skills they need to be successful in adult life because their games are more complex, involve goals and rules, and usually include differentiation of labor.

The school system, curriculum, and teacher expectations continue the gender socialization process by teaching children appropriate gender roles and expectations. Western textbooks contain only limited examples of female role models, women who have made significant contributions to society. As recently as 1977, the ratio of boy-centered stories to girl-centered stories in school textbooks was 7:2 (Tavris & Offir, 1977). This relative lack of role models has had a subtle but significant impact on female socialization.

Research shows contradictory results concerning the comparative abilities of girls and boys in school subjects such as math and verbal and analytical skills. Because of these contradictory results, the author believes that gender differences in intellectual skills can be better explained by gender role socialization and the expectations placed on men and women in society than by biological differences or capabilities.

Gender socialization is not without its costs to both men and women. The high stress level associated with the need to succeed and perform results in higher male mortality rates (Journard, 1974). On the other hand, female passivity and helplessness learned from gender socialization results in a higher incidence of mental illness (Chesler, 1972).

Male and female gender traits do not have to be mutually exclusive in a person's development. Research has shown that female and male college students who score high on both masculine and feminine traits (*i.e.*, androgynous gender role) have higher self-esteem than do students who score high in only one gender role (Spence, Helmreich, & Stapp, 1975). Other research on sex role socialization shows that persons in higher social classes tend to be less rigid about gender distinction and sex role behavior than those in the working and lower classes. Ladner (1971) also reported that black women are socialized to be stronger, more assertive, more self-sufficient, and more independent than white women and to aspire to an occupation. However, black women are also socialized to be nurturing, compassionate, and sensitive.

Recent observation of children in nursery school, however, shows that for the most part traditional female socialization still prevails. Traditional gender socialization of women may result in the following personality traits:

- Problems with self-confidence.
- Lack of trust in themselves and their abilities.
- Underestimation of their own abilities.
- Avoidance of unfamiliar experiences and tasks.
- Lack of resolution when faced with controversy.
- Belief that they are physically weak and vulnerable.
- Inability to communicate easily in front of groups that is rooted in questions about their competence and the value of what they have to say.
- Belief that they are unable to take care of themselves.

It is important to identify these characteristics. Women who believe these characteristics are applicable to themselves act in ways consistent with them and do not attain their full potential. These characteristics are not necessarily true for an individual woman but may significantly hamper that woman's ability to maximize her potential.

Masculine, Feminine, and Androgynous Characteristics

Adults who are strongly motivated to act in a way consistent with traditional male- or female-defined behaviors are considered sex-typed individuals. Adults who are less likely to restrict themselves to traditional masculine or feminine behaviors are considered to have androg-ynous traits. Androgynous persons possess both masculine and femi-nine characteristics and exhibit specific characteristics appropriate to the individual situation (Bem, 1974). They are capable of behaving in either an instrumental (male) or an expressive (female) manner, depending on the specific situation.

Androgyny has its origin in the Latin words *andro* (male) and *gyne* (female). It refers to the joining of masculine and feminine qualities in a single human being. The concept is unsettling to many people, first because it threatens their traditional identity as men or women and, second, because it threatens the security of those who have a vested interest in conventional attitudes toward sex (maleness and female-ness) and gender (masculinity and femininity).

The current societal trend toward androgyny is a result of the same confrontation between masculine and feminine characteristics that caused the women's movement. This movement arose out of grow-ing dissatisfaction with the subordinate role of women in society and attempted to increase freedom and opportunity for women. One of its goals, for example, was to assist women in visualizing themselves as economically independent. Because of the women's movement, the feminine orientation has become more influential in society. This orientation is characterized by the feminine values of cooperation over competition and intuition over rational thinking; it also stresses the importance of relationships over power and violence (Singer, 1976). The increasing acceptance of androgynous characteristics has the potential to liberate people by allowing them to exhibit both masculine and feminine traits rather than limiting them to sex-appropriate characteristics.

Spence and Helmreich (1978) contend that masculinity and femi-ninity are not antithetical characteristics but are independent charac-teristics. They point out that a person may exhibit either strictly masculine or strictly feminine traits, a combination of both types of traits, or a few of each type of trait.

To be an effective professional nurse, a person must be able to exhibit both masculine and feminine characteristics (Flannelly & Flannelly, 1984). This ability to express androgynous characteristics is important for the profession of nursing because the professional nurs-ing role requires humanistic and emotive (feminine) qualities com-bined with a scientific and rational (masculine) approach. To ensure the effectiveness of both the individual nurse and the profession as a whole, nurse educators, managers, and executives must act as role models and demonstrate masculine characteristics such as assertiveness, independence, and intellectual activity as well as the traditional female nurturing characteristics.

Relationship (Dependency) Versus Self (Independence)

The emphasis women place on relationships over self was identified years ago by a number of psychologists, including Helen Deutsch. Deutsch described women as "the ideal life companion" and noted that women were likely to be happiest when they were subordinating themselves to men (Deutsch, 1944). Deutsch went on to report that women were willing to renounce their own achievements for their significant other without feeling they were making a sacrifice. This observation may explain why some women experience significant conflicts when separating from men and attempting to develop their own identities.

Male sex identity and development involves emphatic separation from the mother and individuation; female sex identity is achieved through attachment to others and through identifying and meeting the needs of others. Male gender identity is threatened by intimacy; female gender identity is threatened by separation (Chodorow, 1978).

Kagan and Moss (1962) reported that dependent versus independent traits are formed by the age of three. Boys have traditionally been pushed toward and rewarded for independent behavior, while girls have been encouraged to be dependent on others and not to speak up or physically defend themselves. They have been taught that it is not "ladylike" to fight, that they should depend on a "Prince Charming" to come to their rescue because they do not have enough power to take care of themselves under adverse conditions. This gender socialization has created significant problems in today's society, where women are especially vulnerable to the increase in hostile attacks from men. Bardwick and Douvan (1971) reported that because girls do not experience sufficient stress when they are young, their dependency as adults is encouraged. They do not have adequate practice coping with stressful situations in their early socialization.

The idea of waiting for and relying on Prince Charming to come to the rescue has been described in detail by Dowling (1982), whose thesis is that personal and psychological dependency, or the learned trait of being taken care of by someone else, is the chief factor holding women down. Despite receiving society's permission to achieve significant goals, many women still wait for someone or something external to themselves to transform or rescue them.

Many dependent women marry men they can feel responsible for. This kind of relationship allows the dependent woman to focus all of her attention on her spouse and to avoid looking at herself and her dependency. Other dependent women marry men who have problems such as chemical dependency, alcoholism, the inability to hold down a job, or violent behavior. These women do not acknowledge the problems caused by their spouse's behavior and compensate for the spouse in order to maintain this dependent relationship (Norwood, 1985; Beattie, 1987).

Dependent women have been trained to believe that their husbands are supposed to take care of them physically, economically, and emotionally. When this does not happen in reality, dependent women may conspire to maintain the fantasy that they are taken care of in order to fulfill their dependent needs.

Many women learned as small children that they could usually get what they wanted through dependent behavior. They then learned to control others—fathers, husbands, and children—through their dependent behavior.

Women often enter marriages expecting to conform to the role of wife and mother, while men never expect to change when they get married. This difference contributes to a significant disappointment for many women who expect their husbands will change once married. When dependent women in unhappy marriages finally decide to get a divorce, they often become preoccupied with finding their next husband because they have great difficulty imagining themselves being alone or taking sole responsibility for themselves.

Women who stay in unhappy marriages or jobs they dislike tend to have an unhealthy degree of dependency and a low self-image that inhibits them from separating themselves from the unhappy situation. This difficulty in separating occurs because on an unconscious level they believe they have done something to deserve the misery they are experiencing.

Women have traditionally been taught to avoid taking risks. Parents tend to overprotect their daughters and to communicate that women are vulnerable. This learned belief has put women in a position in which they may have difficulty realizing their full personal and professional potential because they are always "playing it safe."

A number of studies have focused on the role women play in maintaining subordinate thinking and dependency. Social scientists have written about the "female achievement gap," that is, the gap between what females can achieve and what they actually do achieve. Bardwick (1971) identified the unwillingness of many women to assume long-term professional commitments and to seek high-paying careers as two major examples of the ongoing presence of a female achievement gap and the subordinate position of women in society.

The most important factor contributing to dependency in women is the consistently low percentage of women of all ages who believe they must be independent and totally responsible for themselves. Dowling (1982) reported that many women really do not want to be independent and believe it is their right as women to be cared for by others in return for fulfilling the traditional female role. These others include fathers, mothers, husbands, big brothers, children, and bosses.

The truth today, however, is that a majority of women ultimately outlive or are abandoned in some way by those on whom they depend. This is evidenced by the large numbers of widows, displaced home-makers, and divorced women who are heads of households in the early 1990s. Divorce has left many women alone without any skills to support themselves or their children. Death has left many women trying to survive on nothing more than Social Security. Because of the promise that someone else would always be there to take care of them, most of these women have not prepared themselves emotionally or economically to be independent. These women range in age from thirty to fifty-five, and one-third of them are currently living in a state of poverty (Dowling, 1982).

These displaced homemakers tend to have rigid and inflexible personalities and invent a myriad of reasons why they cannot be responsible for themselves. Some of these women may even attempt suicide or use drugs in response to the emotional pain they experience from the loss of the emotional relationships by which they define themselves. Without these relationships, they are lost and have no sense of who they are.

Certain behaviors permit women to maintain their dependent position, including:

- Staying in boring jobs that have no future and poor pay.
- Avoiding asking for raises.
- Reverting to behavior patterns—inability to make decisions for herself, acting helpless, or acting foolish or innocent—that are suitable to "daddy's little girl" rather than to a professional.
- Having children as an excuse to stay home and not pursue career advancement.

Women exhibiting these behaviors usually attribute their situations to numerous factors outside of their control. However, they are the only ones who can change their situation. Leaving an unhappy situation involves risk and pain, but it is easier for them to remain in the miserable situation than to risk taking action.

The disparate visions of the male and female reflect the paradox of the human experience. You learn to know yourself as an individual only after realizing your connection with others. You learn to experience meaningful relationships with others only after you have differentiated yourself from others. These two processes are necessary in order to progress to the maturity of adulthood.

Elizabeth Cady Stanton said in 1848 that self-development is a higher calling than self-sacrifice. Because of their traditional socialization, the greatest conflict for women is between self-development and affiliation with others, responsibility to self as opposed to responsibility to others, and personal rights over the rights of others. The dichotomy between these traditional male and female priorities is shown in Display 1-1.

Maturity for men and women is a process of balancing the rights and responsibilities of others and self. For men, leaving childhood means renouncing relationships in order to develop themselves. For women, leaving childhood means letting go of self and individual freedom to develop and preserve relationships with others (Gilligan, 1982).

External and Internal Loci of Control

Traditional female socialization has focused on an external locus of control rather than an internal one. An external locus of control emphasizes the impact of external factors on an individual's destiny; an internal locus of control emphasizes that factors within an individual are responsible for that person's destiny.

Display 1-1
DICHOTOMY OF MALE AND FEMALE PRIORITIES

Male Priorities	*Female Priorities*
Self	Others
Achievement	Affiliation
Rights	Responsibility
Separation	Connectedness
Selfishness	Self-sacrifice
Identity	Intimacy

When women are successful, they are more likely to attribute their success to luck or to forces external to themselves. Successful men, on the other hand, always take personal credit for their success (Deaux, White, & Farris, 1975). Tavris and Offir (1977) interpreted this to mean that women perceive themselves as more externally controlled, while men think of themselves as more internally controlled.

Matina Horner (1972) described fear of success as one reason many women do not accomplish as much as they are capable of accomplishing. Horner's research showed that some women feel that doing well professionally jeopardizes their relationships with men and that women tend to value their relationships more than success. In 1964, Horner tested the correlation between the actual performance of women and their fear that success would compromise their personal relationships. Her work showed that women who had both high grade-point averages and a high fear of success opted for typical female occupations such as housewife, mother, nurse, and teacher so that their jobs would not threaten their relationships. Horner and Walsh (1974) repeated the study in 1970 to see if the women's movement had had any significant impact on changing women's fear of success. In 1964, she reported, 65% of white women exhibited a positive fear of success; in 1970 that percentage had increased to 88.2%.

The tendency of women to have an external locus of control may help to explain why the profession of nursing has focused most of its efforts to explain and alter its image problems on factors external to the profession and its members. Nurses need to focus on what *they* can do to change their image and the image of the profession. In many instances, they do not believe they have the power to change their image or the profession's by themselves; therefore, they look to external groups for solutions.

As long as women believe that forces external to themselves determine their destinies, thereby putting them in a compromised situation, they do not have to do anything. They can remain preoccupied with fairness issues and do not have to act or to take any responsibility for themselves.

In contrast, successful women have an internal rather than external locus of control. Garfield (1986) identified six attributes commonly found in high performers:

1. Peak performers have missions that motivate them to reach their highest potential.
2. Peak performers attain results in real time and all their activity is directed toward achieving a goal that contributes to their mission.
3. Peak performers use self-management, self-mastery, and the capacity to observe themselves and think effectively.
4. Peak performers are masters in team building and possess an ability to empower others.
5. Peak performers have great mental agility and a high level of concentration.
6. Peak performers anticipate and respond to major changes while maintaining their momentum.

In order to advance themselves and their profession, nurses need to develop strong positive self-images and internal loci of control, as well as the other characteristics listed above, to become peak performers and achievers in the health care industry.

SELF-ESTEEM AND WOMEN

Considerable research has been done on the relationship between self-esteem and performance (Coopersmith, 1967; Rosenberg, 1979). However, nearly all the research has used male subjects. Although there is some contemporary literature that focuses on self-esteem and women, the literature reports clinical observation, case histories, and the personal testimonies of women rather than empirical studies.

Sanford and Donovan (1984) focused on women's self-esteem, assuming four basic premises in their discussions:

1. Low self-esteem in women is largely a result of a male-dominated society.
2. Low self-esteem is the basis for many of the psychological and physical problems that women experience.
3. Low self-esteem in women facilitates low self-esteem in future generations of women.
4. The development of high self-esteem in women is necessary for the future advancement of women as a group.

The Broverman Study (1970) shed some light on the relationship between specific character traits and self-esteem. Seventy-nine mental health professionals were asked to describe specific characteristics of a healthy adult, a healthy male, and a healthy female. Their descriptions of a healthy adult and a healthy male were very similar, and both contrasted sharply with their descriptions of a healthy female.

Much research has also been conducted on the concept of the self-enhancing tendency, which is an individual's tendency to place a high value on the specific traits that person has mastered. Men as a group tend to exhibit this tendency much more frequently than women. For example, if a man has significant scholastic achievements, his scholastic ability plays a very prominent place in the core of his self-concept.

Women, on the other hand, tend to minimize the importance of characteristics they possess and to believe that the traits they feel they lack are more important. For example, if a woman is very competent scholastically, she tends to minimize the importance of scholastic achievements and focuses instead on her perceived inadequacies. The bottom line is that women have been socialized to be humble, to be self-deprecating, and to focus on their weaknesses rather than their strengths.

Pierce (1961) found that high-school-age girls exhibited high achievement motivation regarding success in marriage, attaining personal beauty, social status, and marrying the right man. Because of this high motivation for marriage, the senior year of high school becomes crucial to the success of lower-class girls because it is their

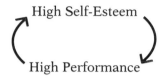

Figure 1-1. High Self-Esteem Performance Cycle

major opportunity or last chance to find a husband. Middle-class girls, on the other hand, experience this pressure in their last year of college because their socioeconomic status allows them to attend school longer (Rubin, 1976). Other societal imperatives have mandated that to be successful, women should have children and should not surpass their husbands' achievements. This socialization has strongly contributed to women's tendency to take temporary jobs rather than pursuing a career.

Cummings (1977) reported that these traditional socialization trends are slowly changing. Women are starting to express greater confidence in themselves and in their ability to combine career, family, and marriage. In our society, status and prestige are associated with monetary rewards that usually result from career achievements. As women focus on careers they can expect status, prestige, and monetary rewards to accompany that changing orientation.

SELF-IMAGE AND PERFORMANCE

Self-image influences behavior and performance in the workplace. It affects how you think and act in the workplace and how you use your work to enhance, preserve, or develop your self-esteem. Self-image can also be a predictor of your occupational choices (Korman, 1966, 1970). Research on the difference between persons with high self-esteem and those with low self-esteem shows:

1. People with high self-esteem are more apt to work harder in response to negative feedback (Brockner & Elkind, 1985).
2. People with high self-esteem are less negatively affected by chronic stressors such as role ambiguity and conflict (Mossholder, Bedian, & Armenakis, 1981).
3. People with high self-esteem are less likely to be affected by acute sources of stress such as workforce layoffs (Brockner, 1988).

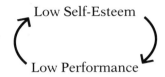

Figure 1-2. Low Self-Esteem Performance Cycle

4. High self-esteem is directly correlated with high job satisfaction (Tharenou, 1979).

There is strong evidence to support a direct and positive relationship between a person's level of self-esteem and that person's achievements (Baruch, 1976; Bedeian & Touliatos, 1978). Women with high self-esteem are more likely to become scientists, physicians, and lawyers; women with lower self-esteem are more likely to become secretaries, teachers, and nurses. High self-esteem increases performance and achievements, which in turn enhance self-esteem.

Low self-esteem, on the other hand, results in lower aspirations, performance, and achievements. When a person achieves at a lower level, that performance reinforces the person's low self-esteem and supports a negative cycle of low performance and self-esteem.

Studies have shown that the father–daughter relationship is very influential in the socialization of successful women (Heilbrun, 1958). When a father encourages his daughter and his approval and love are contingent on her performance, she tends to develop high achievement motivation. High-achieving women tend to be firstborn or only children. They have significant relationships with their fathers, and these relationships are separate and independent from their relationships with their mothers. High-achieving women tend not to be close to their mothers and come from families that do not restrict them to typically female activities. High-achieving women tend to be more independent, assertive, risk-taking, flexible, imaginative, and self-reliant than their peers (Bachtold, 1976; Hennig, 1974; Hoffman, 1972).

SELF-ESTEEM, RELATIONSHIPS, AND SELF

Self-esteem affects more than your feelings about yourself. Rousseau asserted more than two hundred years ago that you cannot love someone else unless you develop a love for yourself (Broome, 1963). You can only relate to and show concern for others to the extent you can relate to and show concern for yourself. Low self-esteem limits a person's ability to relate to others. A positive self-image and a high level of self-esteem permit a person to relate well to others.

Rousseau's assertions have significant implications for the nursing profession. Women usually believe that focusing on themselves is egotistical, unfeminine, selfish, and unhealthy. However, learning to love, respect, and care for yourself is crucial to be able truly to care for and respect your patients and colleagues. A nurse with a low level of self-esteem or concern for self will have a significantly limited capacity to care for others. In the long run, that nurse may become frustrated and burned out because people cannot give something to others that they are unable to give to themselves. To be truly caring professionals, nurses must learn to develop a positive self-image and to care for themselves first.

FEMALE IDENTITY AND EATING DISORDERS

Betty Freidan was the first person to write about eating disorders and female identity (Freidan, 1974). She described the anxiety experienced by women because of the pressure to develop their own identity and independence. Many women had been encouraged to focus most of their attention on home and family and therefore had not learned how to separate themselves from their close association with their mothers. Their struggle to identify their own identities, rather than continuing to live in a role of dependence on their mothers, results in a fixation on food as the symbol of the mother. The woman therefore experiences eating disorders such as overeating and anorexia in her struggle to separate her identity from that of her mother.

Chernin (1981) proposed that the obsession many young women have with food is a response to the anxiety, guilt, and anger they feel over the fact that they can achieve professional goals that their mothers were unable to achieve. Since the 1970s, women have had the opportunity to accomplish almost any goal they set. However, traditional female socialization and the role model provided by the mother can interfere with these opportunities. Chernin proposed that, faced with the pressure and opportunity to be independent, many women feel overwhelmed and unprepared to establish an identity exclusive of their role as daughter, wife, and mother.

Many women have not been encouraged to develop a sense of who they are as individuals outside of their relationships. When placed in a situation in which they are expected to express their personal beliefs and choices, many become confused and feel lost. These feelings represent an identity struggle, and for some this struggle is expressed through a preoccupation with food.

Food represents the dependent tie to the mother. A compulsive preoccupation with food in the form of anorexia, overeating, or bulimia acts out the internal conflict between being like the mother or becoming an independent person. This compulsion with food commands a significant amount of energy and allows women to avoid dealing with the conflict. Ultimately, this inability to separate self from the mother inhibits a woman's ability to grow and establish her independence. In a woman's struggle to find her own identity and to leave behind the traditional dependent identity of the nurturing mother, she may experience a feeling of emptiness, and food is one obsession she may use temporarily to fill that emptiness.

CAREER VERSUS JOB

As mentioned earlier, many women are socialized to believe that if they do the "right" things, there will always be someone to take care of them. As a result, only a small percentage of women prepare themselves for lifelong careers. Many nurses view nursing as a job they can always "fall back on" while awaiting marriage, to subsidize the family income, or to return to when their children are grown. Many women do not visualize themselves as ever being economically self-sufficient.

For these reasons, many nurses view their work as a job rather than a career. Because the differences between a job and a career are significant, this mode of thinking significantly contributes to the present image of the nursing profession.

People who are engaged in a career are motivated first to make a contribution and second to make a living. Career-motivated people frequently relate that they would continue in their chosen work irrespective of the economic incentives offered. On the other hand, people

n jobs are primarily working for the economic incentives.
ivated people have a long-term focus. They are usually sala-
o not focus on the hours they work, while people in jobs
ocus on the specific number of hours they work and the
nou..,   es they are paid.

These differing attitudes toward a job and a career significantly affect the ability of nursing to acquire professional status. As long as a majority of nurses see nursing as a short-term job undertaken to meet their economic needs, and as long as they focus on hourly wage rates rather than considering what they need to do to make a contribution to the profession, nursing will have difficulty acquiring professional status.

SOCIALIZATION OF NURSES

Historically, women who nursed the sick came from the lower classes. The Florence Nightingale image of the nurse that developed in the Victorian Era was an attempt to upgrade the stereotype of the nurse to one who could act like a lady and endure the challenges of nursing those injured in war.

The technical and intellectual component of curing the sick was differentiated from the emotional component of caring for the sick. As a result of traditional gender socialization and beliefs about male and female traits and abilities, men were assigned the intellectual component of curing, that is, the profession of medicine, while women were relegated to the expressive component of caring for the sick, that is, nursing (Clark, 1986).

If gender socialization and the traditional socialization of nurses are combined, the following messages for nurses result:

1. Good nurses always consider the patients' and physicians' needs before their own.
2. Good nurses always anticipate the needs of physicians and patients.
3. Good nurses are totally responsible for the well-being of patients and physicians.
4. Good nurses always treat physicians with the highest respect, never question their judgment, and anticipate their every need without coming across as being too smart or challenging.

5. Good nurses always follow policies and procedures and never take shortcuts or become innovative.
6. Good nurses always follow directions from senior nurses rather than thinking for themselves.

Throughout the history of the profession, a number of stereotypes about nurses have also developed that need to be acknowledged and challenged by nurses who desire to be taken seriously in their careers. The stereotypes are listed and briefly discussed here.

1. The nurse as a woman in white who represents virtue, purity, and virginity. These traits have no connection with the attributes of a professional or a nurse. The nurse's cap is also a remnant of the female's need to cover her head to show subservience and is rooted in religious custom.
2. The nurse as a torturer. This stereotype has been exhibited in cartoons and get-well cards that depict nurses attacking patients with huge syringes and enema bags.
3. The nurse as a sex symbol. This stereotype has pervaded media depictions of nurses.
4. The nurse as a handmaid for the physician. This stereotype is still prevalent in hospitals, although it is slowly changing. It is documented as the main cause of stress and frustration for nurses who provide direct patient care in hospitals.
5. The nurse as battle-ax. This stereotype has largely been used by physicians to denote nurses who have been promoted through advanced education, assertiveness, and career planning to the role of nurse manager or nurse executive. Assertiveness and independent interpersonal skills are frequently interpreted by physicians and other nurses as overly aggressive, unfeminine traits.
6. The "clipboard" nurse. As nurse managers become more successful and effective in their leadership roles, there is a shift in the stereotype from the battle-ax supervisor to the "clipboard" nurse who does nothing but check clipboards and do useless paperwork. When these nurses have to return to their white uniforms and care for patients, physicians become more comfortable with them and make comments such as, "It's good to see you working today," or "I hate to see all the good nurses go into management where they don't do anything important."

Although in the 1990s some nurses seek individuation and autonomy, many exhibit ambivalence and anxiety in pursuing these goals. They usually respond to this anxiety and ambivalence through denial, projection, inappropriate expressions of anger, and a dissociation from peers (Byrne, 1982). These are coping mechanisms that all people use at one time or another when establishing identities separate from their parents. Traditional male socialization encouraged this separation at an early age, when boys typically have the support and encouragement of their parents to separate. Women typically struggle with this separation after they leave home and exhibit these behaviors in the workplace.

Those female nurses who fail to escape from their socialized dependency to a new independent existence project their dependency onto others and blame them for their situation and circumstances. As long as nurses continue to use projection and to blame external factors for their situation, they will remain dependent because they will not take responsibility for their lives. Because they are unable to take responsibility for their situation, they never take action. Projection may be one of the biggest reasons that women and nurses stay in their traditional secondary position. As long as nurses focus their energy on blaming others—parents, husbands, teachers, bosses, hospital administrators, or physicians—they will not take responsibility for their situation, nor will they take positive action to improve it.

A second way many nurses respond to their struggle for independence is to deny their anger and frustration. Most men have learned that it is acceptable to express anger and then to get over it. Therefore, they are able to express anger one minute and socialize with the person they were angry with the next minute. Many women, on the other hand, tend to deny their anger and to "keep score." When their anger becomes overwhelming, they either lose control or develop deep-seated resentments toward the person. This repression of anger and build-up of resentment result in feelings of helplessness, victimization, and depression that can lead to physical and emotional problems (Symonds, 1976).

It is important to assist nurses in identifying, understanding, and changing their self-images and self-limiting behaviors. When nurses can recognize the consequences of their socialized thinking, they can change their thoughts and their beliefs about themselves. This change permits them in turn to change their actions, performance, and achievements.

Examples of nonproductive behavior that has been observed in nurses by the author include the following:

- When communicating with physicians, nurses often add tag phrases to their assessments, such as "Don't you agree?" or "I may be wrong, but. . . ." This pattern of communication results from a lack of confidence in their ability in relation to that of the physician. By their words, they are acknowledging the subordinate position that they resent.
- Many nurses refer their problems to their supervisors because they are not comfortable communicating negative issues directly with peers, colleagues, and physicians. They have learned that it is acceptable to take their problems to an authority figure, and they believe that they do not have the power, authority, or skills to deal with the conflict or controversy themselves.
- A significant number of nurses are married to abusive or chemically dependent men. These nurses usually hide such problems from their families, friends, and employers and tend to withdraw from others. They feel that they are responsible for their problems and should be able to fix them, and that to be a good wife means to persevere. They believe that they have no other options, and subconsciously they believe they deserve this kind of life. They take responsibility for their spouses' behavior and frequently work two jobs or a significant amount of overtime to compensate for their irresponsible and per-haps unemployed spouses. In some cases, they divorce their chemi-cally dependent husbands only to marry others who have the same problem.
- A high divorce rate has been observed among nurses. This personal failure may magnify a nurse's existing low self-image. In other instances, nurses may marry persons who have problems, but whom they feel they can "fix" or turn around because they are nurses.
- A significant number of nurses (and physicians) have chemical dependency problems themselves. As previously mentioned, women have traditionally been protected from stressful situations beginning in childhood through their relationships with stronger protectors. As professional nurses, they are faced with high-stress situations for which they are not prepared. Because of nurses' proximity to drugs and their relationships with physician prescribers, they have easy access to drugs to assist them in coping with stressful work or home situations.

- A higher percentage of nurses have weight problems than do other female professionals. This problem is heightened by the expectation that medical professionals should be good role models for health and fitness.

NURSING'S STRUGGLE FOR PROFESSIONAL IDENTITY

A number of articles on nursing have discussed the profession's struggle to separate and individuate itself from the field of medicine.

Mahler (1979) described the struggle to separate and individuate from the mother as a second birth that results in a regression to a state of negativism or progression to a state of adolescence. Rodgers (1981), following Mahler, described nursing's separation/individuation as a struggle to separate from the medical profession and establish individual and professional identity away from authority figures. This struggle for separation is magnified by the fact that the medical profession is male dominated.

Rodgers explains that some nurses who are struggling through this separation regress to earlier phases of negativism and dependency because they wish to maintain their symbiotic relationship with physicians. This behavior can be seen in nurses who solicit support from physicians to represent them and speak on their behalf rather than dealing directly with the administration. However, the desire to maintain this symbiotic relationship with the medical profession is for some nurses accompanied by strong feelings of anger and frustration over the need to be dependent. These conflicting feelings may be exhibited in militant self-sufficiency or pseudo-independence. Nurses who progress through separation usually temporarily exhibit typical adolescent behavior, or a black-or-white, right-or-wrong mind-set. Eventually, they progress through this adolescent behavior to a more adult, assertive behavior pattern.

Men and women tend to experience the separation process very differently. Men tend to separate by aggressive, delinquent acts; women tend to remain subservient or to separate by typical adolescent behavior (Rodgers, 1981). If women remain subservient, they assume the helper role for physicians. If they choose adolescent behavior, they usually emphasize their sexuality through flirting behavior or exhibit anger or argumentative characteristics. They progress through this period by focusing on what they are against rather than what they are for. However, this eventually allows them to define who they are. Over time, adolescent or subservient behavior may be replaced by assertive adult behavior.

Roberts (1983) used the model of oppressed groups to discuss the problems of nursing. In this model, the dominant group has the ability to identify its norms and values as the correct norms and values for society. These norms give that group power over the subordinate group or groups within the society. Members of the subordinate group who wish to accomplish their goals try to assimilate the behavior patterns of the dominant group. These people are in turn classified as "marginal" individuals because they are on the fringes of both the dominant and the subordinate groups. The internalization of dominant-group behavior by the marginal person leads to self-hatred and low self-esteem. The subordinate group, in turn, develops aggressive feelings that cannot be expressed to the dominant group and that result in the expression of anger through passive-aggressive behavior patterns. This inability to attack the dominant group is also expressed through horizontal violence, or fighting among members within the subordinate group. Roberts believes that many nurses exhibit self-hatred, a dislike of other nurses, and a lack of self-esteem.

There is another side to the separation equation: the parent figure may have difficulty allowing the child to separate. Just as some parents keep their children tied to them on some level, there are examples of the medical profession's reluctance to let the nursing profession go out on its own. A recent example of this reluctance is the proposal by the American Medical Association to introduce registered care technicians, to assist nursing in meeting its obligation to care for patients in hospitals. The registered care technician proposal introduced an alternative health care worker controlled by physicians to care for patients in the absence of the appropriate nursing staff in hospitals.

On a positive note, nurses and physicians who can relate on a collegial level without feeling threatened have made the transition to adulthood and possess a high level of self-esteem (Rodgers, 1981). Successful separation into the role of adult results in the ability to assume total responsibility for the self. Successful individuation eliminates the need to place blame on others, to provide excuses for one's shortcomings, or to feel oneself to be a victim.

Accomplishing this separation/individuation is important for nurses and for the profession as a whole. Nurses who fail to undergo this process experience a sense of alienation and frustration. To rid the profession of this frustration and alienation, nurses need to make this transition to independence. They must develop positive professional self-images and assist their colleagues to do the same.

The traditional socialization undergone by women and by nurses can explain some of the frustration and image problems of the profession today. Understanding the impact of this traditional socialization is a first step nurses must take in order to realize that this process can be reversed. When individual nurses understand how their thinking has been affected by their socialization, they can in turn take action to resocialize themselves and become anything they choose to be. They can take charge of their own personal and professional lives by developing a positive and professional self-image and by enhancing their performance to achieve great things.

2

Self-Image Models and the Nursing Profession

The more computers are understood and used, the more they are compared to the brain. In fact, the brain operates in a way very similar to a computer. The brain stores millions of bits of information that have been programmed into it throughout a person's life. Daily experiences are "inputted" into the brain and stored in memory similar to the way data are key-punched into computers and stored.

Some of the data that have been inputted into a person's brain are accurate and valid, while some are not. All information is nevertheless saved in the brain as if it were true. All our behavior and actions in turn are driven by the data that have been inputted into the brain in the form of thoughts and beliefs, whether these thoughts and beliefs are true or not. Figure 2-1 (p. 31) outlines specific factors affecting the thoughts and beliefs stored in the brain that determine self-image or the picture we have of ourselves and our behavior and performance.

This chapter discusses three models that describe how self-image is developed and how it determines a person's behavior, actions, performance, and achievements. The specific assumptions and principles of each model will be described in detail within the context of professional nursing.

KEY CHAPTER CONCEPTS

Key Concept #1

Personal experiences, heredity, environment, gender socialization, and reference groups influence your thoughts and beliefs about who you are.

Key Concept #2

Thoughts and beliefs determine your self-image.

Key Concept #3

All your behavior, actions, and performance are consistent with your self-image.

Key Concept #4

Your conscious mind acts as a servomechanism to actualize what your subconscious mind believes to be true about you.

Key Concept #5

Your level of performance and achievement is directly related to your ability to assume total responsibility for yourself. This ability, in turn, is directly related to your self-image.

Key Concept #6

The image of the nursing profession is directly related to the self-image of individual nurses.

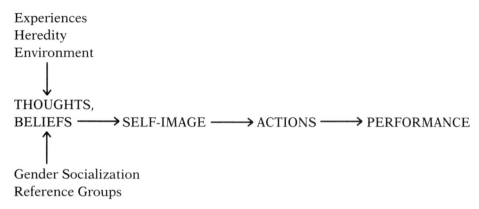

Figure 2-1. Factors Determining Individual Thoughts, Beliefs, Self-Image, Actions, and Performance

THE SELF-IMAGE MODEL

Psychologists such as Carl Rogers (1961) have described the self-image as a composite of the thoughts and beliefs people hold about themselves or the picture of the person they believe themselves to be *(Key Concept #2)*. Personal experiences, heredity, environment, gender socialization, and reference groups influence our thoughts and beliefs about who we are *(Key Concept #1)*. Our thoughts and beliefs are a product of gender socialization, past experiences, triumphs, failures, and other people's reactions and perceptions of us.

As a result of these influences, we develop a picture of ourselves, or a self-image, which we believe to be true in all respects. In reality, this picture can be distorted and can contain some characteristics that are not true. Nevertheless, our self-image is true for us because we *believe* it is true. Because of this belief, we always act in accordance with our self-image because we cannot consistently act differently from what we believe to be true *(Key Concept #3)*.

A number of studies have identified people whose childhood experiences have convinced them that they were not as intelligent as other children. As a result of this belief, these people developed a poor self-image and acted and performed as though they were less intelligent than other children. Later in life, tests have shown that these people had normal capabilities. This new information changed their thoughts and beliefs about themselves, thereby also changing their performance and achievements.

The development of self-image occurs in childhood and adolescence (Rosenberg, 1979). Coopersmith (1967) identified a number of factors that are positively associated with the development of a positive self-image in children. These factors include: (1) the self-image of the mother; (2) the marital adjustment of the parents; (3) the mother's perception of the child's intelligence; (4) the mother's affection for the child and the quality of the rapport between them.

When people participate in the workforce, their self-image is affected by a number of other factors (Kohn & Schooler, 1983; Korman, 1970). These factors can be divided into intrinsic job characteristics and external job characteristics. Intrinsic job characteristics that are positively correlated with high employee self-image include job variety, a high level of skill, content of job, employee participation in decision-making about the job, and low role strain.

Employees with positive self-images tend to have an internal locus of control, whereas employees with poor self-images are more externally controlled. Internally controlled employees believe that they can make an impact on the organization; externally controlled employees perceive that they are controlled by the organization (Dweck, 1975). The self-image and self-esteem of externally driven people within organizations is also a function of self-comparison. In other words, these people expect to move up in the organization, and they compare their current self with their former self in relation to their specific expectations about their performance and their jobs. Their self-image and self-esteem can be affected negatively or positively according to how their perception of their position or role in the organization compares with their expectations.

The influence of an external versus internal locus of control is very important in developing plans to improve the quality of work and environment of the professional nurse. When a majority of nurses are externally motivated, it takes more than external organizational changes to improve their perception of their workplace and worklife. Interventions to change nurses' perceptions of their power base and influence must be implemented to make significant changes to enhance their performance.

THE PSYCHOCYBERNETIC MODEL

The psychocybernetic model also articulates that self-image determines performance. Maltz (1975), a plastic surgeon, developed the term "psychocybernetics" in his book of the same name. Maltz reported that unattractive people tended to act unattractive and to perform poorly because they had poor self-images. However, after undergoing plastic surgery to improve their physical appearance, many of these people still exhibited behavior consistent with a poor self-image and did not appear to be happier or more successful than prior to their surgery. Maltz concluded that self-image determines how people behave and perform in all situations. Therefore, he proposed that any attempts to improve a person's performance, quality of life, and overall happiness need to include interventions to enhance the person's self-image. Because all our behavior and actions are driven by our beliefs about ourselves, all attempts to improve the performance and quality of life must include developing a positive self-image that is consistent with being a happy and successful person.

Psychocybernetics combines principles from the fields of psychology and cybernetics. The science of cybernetics concerns teleology, or the goal-striving operation of mechanical systems. Cybernetics explains how a mechanical system is programmed to reach a specific goal and stems from the work of physicists and mathematicians (Maltz, 1975).

Maltz followed the lead of Prescott Lecky, a pioneer in self-image psychology, in reporting that personality and behavior are determined by the mental and spiritual picture we hold of ourselves. The brain and nervous system function as a servomechanism or goal-striving mechanism, to actualize a person's self-image. The conscious mind acts as a servomechanism to actualize what the subconscious mind believes to be true about the person *(Key Concept #4)*. If a person has a positive self-image, the brain directs that person to accomplish significant goals. On the other hand, if a person has a negative or poor self-image, the brain directs that person's body to actualize failure behavior. Figures 2-2 and 2-3 illustrate how the brain functions as a servomechanism to actualize the goals it believes to be true. In each of these situations the brain, as a servomechanism, directs the body and mind to do what needs to be done on an unconscious level to actualize the traits the person believes to be true about the self.

There are two major principles that determine the impact self-image has on a person's life as a result of the servomechanism of the brain. First, everything we do is consistent with our self-image *(Key Concept #3)*. In other words, we always act like the person we believe ourselves to be. As a result of the servomechanistic nature of the brain, we literally are incapable of acting differently from our self-image. Self-image functions like a software program to direct all our physical

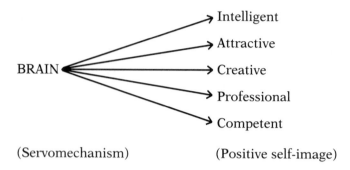

(Servomechanism)   (Positive self-image)

Figure 2-2. How the Brain Actualizes a Positive Self-Image

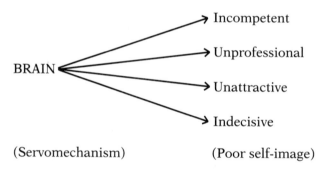

(Servomechanism)   (Poor self-image)

Figure 2-3. How the Brain Actualizes a Poor Self-Image

and emotional actions and behavior. This program or servomechanism is results- or outcome-oriented. Self-image is buried in the subconscious mind, and the conscious mind does what needs to be done in order to actualize that self-image. If one has the self-image of a person who has problems, is a victim, or is unlucky, that person's brain will direct physical, emotional, and mental faculties on a subconscious level to actualize that picture. On the other hand, if a person has the self-image of being a winner, being in control, and being successful and intelligent, that person's brain will direct all its faculties to do what needs to be done to actualize that self-image.

If, as a nurse, you have the self-image of being a victim, not appreciated, and subordinate to physicians, your actions will act out that self-image. Despite the fact that you may dislike these characteristics in other nurses, if you believe they are true about yourself, your body and mind will act in accordance with them all of the time.

If you believe that you are not in control of your nursing practice or feel you have no input into the functioning of your department, you will behave in ways that are consistent with those beliefs. No matter how much control or authority you are actually given, you will not see it and will not take advantage of it because you don't believe you have that power.

Self-image is originally developed through a person's thoughts, experiences, environment, and reference groups. Therefore, by changing our thoughts, experiences, environment, and reference groups, we can reprogram our self-image from negative to positive, as well as from positive to negative. This reprogramming process is covered in later chapters.

The second major principle influencing self-image is simply stated: If you can think it, you can attain it. This principle, which supports *Key Concepts #2* and *#3,* means that if any idea, thought, or belief enters your mind, you literally have the mental, emotional, and physical ability to accomplish it. The only factors that stand between you and your dreams and goals are hard work, a willingness to take risks, and perseverance.

This principle opens many doors for some people; however, it creates significant anxiety for others. Some people are threatened by it because it puts total responsibility for success on their own shoulders and eliminates the option of giving excuses or placing blame on others and on circumstances. When one understands and embraces this principle, that person can no longer blame external factors for successes or failures. Some people, however, are more comfortable going through life feeling helpless, unlucky, or not intelligent enough to accomplish their dreams. It is easier and less risky than acknowledging that they have the ability and responsibility to accomplish whatever they really desire.

COMPONENTS OF THE MIND

The mind is divided into the subconscious mind and the conscious mind. The subconscious mind is the servomechanism, or program, that contains your self-image. The subconscious mind holds all the programs that have been put into you throughout your life. Those programs cannot be erased and will always be a part of you. However, additional or alternative programs can be put into the subconscious mind at any time.

The subconscious mind operates much more quickly or automatically than the conscious mind. When a person is in a particular situation that requires an immediate response, the subconscious mind plugs into one of its existing programs automatically. For example, if you are driving down the freeway and another car pulls out in front of you, your subconscious mind plays the tape you learned in driving school to put on the brakes and swerve to avoid the car.

Programs enter the subconscious mind through socialization, repetition, or a significant emotional event. Therefore, although a person cannot erase a negative program put into the subconscious mind during childhood socialization, revised or additional programs can be put into the subconscious mind through the use of repetition. Chapters three through six outline specific methods of reprogramming the subconscious mind to enhance personal and professional self-image.

The conscious mind implements the overall direction set by the subconscious mind. The conscious mind only pays attention to factors in one's environment and experience that are consistent with the person's self-image. External factors or opportunities that are inconsistent with what the subconscious mind believes to be true are ignored or screened out by the conscious mind, whereas external factors and opportunities that are consistent with self-image receive attention and action.

It has been reported that in contemporary society, a person may be bombarded by 350 to 700 messages per day. These messages are communicated by television, radio, newspapers, professional journals, advertisements, fellow employees, significant others, superiors, subordinates, etc. In order to process all this information, people develop screens to filter and sort it. The criteria by which information is screened or sorted are based on the person's self-image. These screens allow information to be absorbed that is consistent with a person's perceived interests, abilities, and goals.

These screens are constructed based on personal and professional self-image. For example, if you have a professional self-image of a staff nurse who is not interested in or capable of becoming a nurse manager, you will screen out advertisements for nurse manager positions, continuing education, or university education geared to nurse managers, and will not respond to colleagues who encourage you to

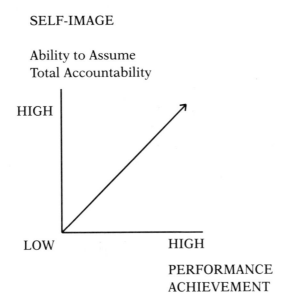

                        ABILITY TO TAKE   PERFORMANCE
SELF-IMAGE ———→ TOTAL RESPONSIBILITY ———→ ACHIEVEMENT
                        FOR SELF

Figure 2-4. Tracy's Achievement Model I

SELF-IMAGE

Ability to Assume
Total Accountability

HIGH

LOW   HIGH

                              PERFORMANCE
                              ACHIEVEMENT

Figure 2-5. Tracy's Achievement Model II

apply for a nurse manager position. You will not even be aware of these possibilities in your environment.

THE PSYCHOLOGY OF ACHIEVEMENT

Tracy proposed that individual achievement is a function of one's willingness and ability to take full responsibility and accountability for one's personal and professional life, which he theorized is directly related to self-image (Tracy, 1986). Figures 2-4 and 2-5 show two ways of displaying the relationship between self-image, the ability to assume total responsibility for one's life, and performance and achievement.

This is an important concept for nurses. One of the major concerns for the profession is that many nurses do not feel in control of their practices and feel helpless and frustrated. According to Tracy's model, the feeling of being in control is directly related to having a positive self-image. The feeling of being in control or having the power to influence one's environment is a function of a positive self-image rather than of a specific environment, organization, or situation. Nurses historically have focused their frustration of not feeling in control on external rather than internal factors.

Tracy's model shows that as a nurse, you are responsible for your own feelings of being in control. No person or external factor can give you that feeling. You can only acquire it after you develop a strong positive self-image and realize that you are completely responsible for your situation. There may be external factors and environments that are very stifling and negative. However, as an adult and a professional responsible for your own destiny, you can choose to remove yourself from those factors. A positive self-image can help get you into an environment that will support your definition of success.

Blaming external factors encourages one to look for outside solutions rather than taking action. Action only comes after one comes to the realization that one is totally responsible for, accountable for, and able to change the circumstances of personal and professional life that one is unhappy with.

The implications of this model are dramatic for nurses and nurse administrators. Organizational attempts to assist nurses to feel more in control of their practices through reorganization, giving them more power and input into policy formulation, and improving recognition and reward mechanisms will not be effective if the nurses have poor self-images. The only action that allows nurses to feel in control is assuming total responsibility for their own professional practice through the development of a positive professional self-image. This may explain why many nurses still perceive themselves as powerless despite the significant reorganizational changes and salary adjustments that have been made in many health care organizations in the early 1990s.

Tracy's model shows that programs aimed at improving the self-image of nurses can be effective in changing the image and achievements of the profession. Although many nurses express a desire for professional status and image, some have not been able to internalize the thoughts and beliefs that drive professionals. Therefore, their actions and behavior are not those of professionals. Typical examples of such behavior include:

1. Aggressive, compensatory actions
2. Giving excuses for professional problems
3. Blaming behavior
4. Risk-averse actions
5. Lack of healthy role-modeling behavior
6. Nonprofessional appearance and dress
7. Preoccupation with hourly wage rates and overtime pay
8. Avoiding involvement in peer review
9. Not seeking higher education.

Tracy described worry as the process of negative goal-setting. When a person is preoccupied with events, conditions, or goals that the person wishes to avoid, the subconscious mind actually internalizes these events, conditions, or goals and the conscious mind acts to realize them. The mind cannot actualize a negative concept. It merely instructs the body to actualize a person's mental images or thoughts.

There are four strategies for avoiding the stress, strain, and negative programming influences of worry. First, define the exact situation or thing that worries you. Worrying often results from fear of the unknown. In most cases, when you specifically define what you are worried about, the fear and anxiety will disappear. People often worry about things that will never happen, and yet their bodies and minds pay the price because they experience the stress of the situation through worrying.

Second, identify the worst possible consequence of the situation you fear. In most cases, you will realize that it is not as bad as you feared. This process allows you to put your fear into perspective and to realize that what you fear is actually not the worst thing that could happen to you.

Third, resolve in your mind to accept the worst-case scenario if it should occur.

Fourth, identify an action that you can take to avoid the worst-case scenario. By taking action, you will not feel as if the situation is controlling you and that you are helpless. By being proactive, you turn the situation around, and feel that you have some power over it. If the worst-case scenario actually occurs, you will be mentally prepared to accept it and go on.

There are a number of things people do on a daily basis to program themselves to actualize negative outcomes that they would not voluntarily choose to actualize. These behaviors and thinking patterns are learned through socialization. People need to be aware of them and to take steps to avoid them in their daily lives in order to maximize their performance and enhance the quality of their lives.

There are some actions that must be taken to avoid negative programming. First, never say negative things about yourself because you will actually program yourself to make these things come true. For example, if you say to your friends or family, "I'll never be able to finish this task," you are actually programming your subconscious mind to believe that you cannot do it, and you will not be able to accomplish the task. When you question your ability to perform in a particular role—saying, for example, "I'll never be able to go back to school to get my graduate degree," or "I'm just not good with numbers"—you are in fact programming yourself to actualize that outcome. You may very well have the capability to fulfill the role, but negative thinking will convince your subconscious self-image that you are unable to accomplish the goal.

Second, never say something about yourself to others or to yourself that you do not actually want to happen. For example, if you say to yourself that you know you will never be able to get along with a particular person, you in fact will never be able to get along with that person because your mind and body will act on an unconscious level to maintain a conflict situation with that person. Conscious efforts to get along with that person will be sabotaged in order to maintain your preprogrammed tape of not getting along with the person.

Third, do not let others motivate or control you, and do not motivate others, through guilt or blaming. Separate yourself from environments in which guilt and blaming occur because it is very likely that you will internalize the guilt that you encounter. For example, if a superior tells you often enough that you need to compensate for specific inadequacies, you will soon believe that you have significant inadequacies, whether you really do or not. If you believe that you are inadequate in some areas, your behavior and actions will be consistent with that belief and you will allow yourself to be manipulated by information that may not be true.

Fourth, learn to forgive and forget past hurts. If you do not, you will carry anger, resentment, and frustration with you that ultimately will interfere with your happiness and performance. Over time, deep-seated resentments toward this person or persons may build up, and you may develop a victim mentality. If you begin to believe that you are a victim, you will begin to behave like a victim. Over time, this behavior and the accompanying consequences can become a way of life.

According to Tracy, the first people that need to be forgiven for past transgressions are a person's parents (Tracy, 1986). Everyone has suffered perceived injustices at the hands of their parents. Some people believe that their parents treated them unfairly, were too strict or too lenient, did not love them, abused them, abandoned them, etc. Some people resent being part of a large family, while others resent being an only child. The specific issues do not matter. The important thing is how people react to their perceptions of what happened to them. To become a mature adult, people must acknowledge that their parents did the best job they could in raising them and must give up any past resentments they have been harboring. This forgiveness can be accomplished by developing and repeating a positive affirmation such as: "I forgive you, mom and dad, completely for everything I was ever upset about."

People cannot truly relate to others as adults until they give up deep-seated resentments and relate to their parents as adults. Parents are a person's first and most important role models and authority figures. Many employees in the workplace have significant difficulty relating to their superiors as a direct result of their inability to develop an adult relationship with their parents by giving up deep-seated resentments.

SELF-IMAGE AND HEALTH

Siegel (1989) states that a chronic belief in and feeling of helplessness has significant physical ramifications for people. He reports that the chronic feeling of not being in control of self depletes the brain of the vital neurotransmitter norepinephrine, the chemical in the brain that is necessary for feelings of happiness and contentment.

People who feel in control of their lives can withstand enormous amounts of change and still thrive. People who do not feel in control of their lives are physically and emotionally drained by the same changes and challenges.

The feeling of being in control is first learned by the infant through interactions with significant others. Later in life, the external factors of environment, socialization, and reference groups either support or destroy this feeling. Siegel contends that when people learn helplessness from their environment, they develop depressed personalities and feelings of defeatism. When they believe they have no control, they act in ways that are consistent with that belief and act out this helplessness.

Kobasa compared people who developed a condition of helplessness with those who developed a condition of hardiness, or the ability to overcome helplessness. She found three basic attitudes that described the hardy personality: (1) commitment or involvement; (2) control, or the belief that the individual could influence events around him; and (3) challenge, or the belief that life changes stimulate growth rather than being a threat to the status quo. Kobasa called this transformational coping, as opposed to regressive coping (cited in Siegel, 1989).

Vaillant (1979) reported that mental health is the most important predictor of physical health. Therefore, a person's self-programming affects not only performance and achievements but also physical health. Siegel reported numerous studies that showed that people with positive self-images seemed to be healthier, avoided debilitating diseases, and dealt more effectively with physical and mental illnesses than did people with poor self-images. It is known that people are more susceptible to disease when they are under emotional stress than when they are confident and goal-directed. A wide range of illnesses, including high blood pressure, headaches, ulcers, allergies, heart disease, and digestive disease, are strongly associated with anxiety and stress reactions (Siegel, 1989).

As a health care professional, it is crucial for you to be engaged in active, positive programming of your own life in order to be good physical and emotional role models for your patients and fellow professionals.

SELF-IMAGE AND
SELF-ACTUALIZATION

An important concept in the discussion of self-image and self-esteem was identified by the noted psychologist Abraham Maslow. Maslow

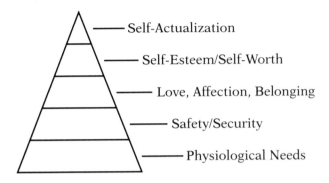

Figure 2-6. Maslow's Hierarchy of Needs

developed a model that describes a hierarchy of common needs motivating all persons (Figure 2-6).

According to Maslow's model, people seek to become self-actualized, or the best they can be. In order for people to attain their highest potential, however, their lower-level needs must be met in the order in which they appear in the hierarchy. Therefore, a person's potential cannot be fulfilled until the needs for self-esteem and self-worth are satisfied. Everyone knows people that appear to be stuck on one of the lower levels of Maslow's hierarchy of needs, inhibiting them from attaining their full potential in their personal and professional lives.

Self-actualization describes personal and professional growth through individual effort and action. It does not mean that a person has attained perfection. Self-actualization means that the person has arrived at personally selected life goals that operationalize that person's true potential. A person's true potential can only be defined when that person can see and value the unique talents, abilities, and inclinations that come through the development of a positive self-image.

A positive self-image is not to be confused with narcissistic pride or a big ego. People who have a positive or healthy self-image are in touch with and accept their strengths and weaknesses. Conversely, people who are not in touch with their strengths and weaknesses usually have poor self-images and need to compensate for their feelings of inferiority by emphasizing their strengths, bragging about their accomplishments, or criticizing others to bring them down to their perceived level. People with positive self-images, however, accept their liabilities as well as their assets and can speak about both in realistic terms.

The process of reaching one's full potential through the development of a positive self-image also requires developing a sense of responsibility for oneself. The word "responsibility" in this context is defined as the ability to respond positively and proactively to situations that occur in one's life rather than rationalizing or blaming external forces or other people. All people face choices in life, and being responsible adults requires them to take action by making appropriate choices to respond to their environment in order to fulfill their potential.

All people face difficult, unfortunate, and challenging situations in the course of their lives. A characteristic of the successful person, or the winner, is the ability to respond positively to challenging and sometimes unfortunate events. Successful people often have more unfortunate things happen to them than unsuccessful people do. However, they are able to rise above difficult times and respond in a responsible manner, communicating that they will pick themselves up and start over again. It has been said many times that it is not what happens to a person that counts, it is how the person responds that separates the winners from the losers.

Unsuccessful people tend to be immobilized by challenges and unfortunate situations. They tend to react to these challenges by rationalization, complaining about how unfair the world is or how unlucky they are. They tend to "play it safe," avoiding future challenges or unhappy, unsuccessful situations.

People with positive self-images also tend to relate to others with respect, kindness, and dignity, whereas people with low self-images attempt to bring others down to their level and to try to take advantage of them. Learning to value oneself is critical to attaining one's highest potential and relating to others in a positive and meaningful way.

A positive self-image can be developed by anyone, regardless of past difficult experiences. People have the power within themselves to choose happiness over unhappiness, self-fulfillment over self-defeat, and hope over despair. However, people who maintain a negative self-image give up their personal power to be self-fulfilled and choose to be victims of their environment. They focus on luck and chance as the forces determining their position in the world rather than choosing to take full responsibility for their own self-fulfillment and self-actualization.

SELF-IMAGE AND CODEPENDENCY

Much has been written in the contemporary literature about the personality trait of codependency. Codependency is described as the tendency to be addicted to misery. This personality characteristic is prevalent in people who have chronically poor self-images and who perceive themselves to be inadequate and worthless.

An addiction is defined as a compulsion or obsession for something that in turn creates problems in one's life. As a result of the belief that they deserve to be miserable, codependents believe that they need to play the roles of rescuer and savior in dysfunctional relationships or situations. They actually assume the role of victim and scapegoat ultimately to maintain their source of misery. Codependent persons choose to stay in miserable situations and provide many reasons why they cannot leave these situations. Behavior characteristics that codependents exhibit include:

1. They deny that the addiction is creating problems in their lives.
2. They lose control of themselves and everything around them as a result of their behavior.
3. They continue to stay in situations that create significant problems for them and believe that they have no other choice.
4. They generally repress their feelings about their miserable situation.
5. They have constant obsessive and compulsive thoughts about their situation but do not and cannot take action to remove themselves from the situation.
6. They have withdrawal symptoms such as anxiety attacks when they are not experiencing the misery or crises that they are used to. When things temporarily improve, they become suspicious and feel that they are being set up for bigger problems.

Codependency ultimately represents the chronic behavior of people with chronic poor self-images. The condition can be eliminated by drastically improving the person's self-image.

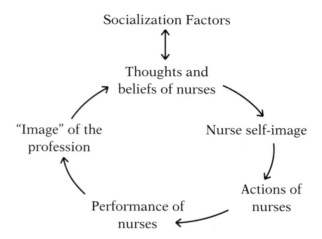

Figure 2-7. Relationship of Individual Nurses to the Image of Nursing

APPLYING THE SELF-IMAGE MODEL
TO NURSING

The self-image model is very useful in explaining the factors that affect the thoughts, beliefs, performance, and achievements of nurses, which in turn affect the overall performance and achievements of the profession. Figure 2-7 illustrates how the image of the profession is affected by the thoughts and beliefs of individual nurses.

Display 2-1 (pp. 48–49) outlines some of the historical factors that have determined the thoughts and beliefs of individual nurses. Historically, society believed that nursing was not a very challenging career and that the average woman could be a good nurse. Some people believed that all one had to do to be a good nurse was to be nurturing and to follow the physician's orders. It was believed that the medical profession did all the difficult thinking and decision-making. Applying the self-image model, these ideas were learned through environmental factors, traditional female socialization, and the reference groups that historically programmed nurses.

The nursing profession has been struggling for professional status. In many instances, the thinking, beliefs, and actions of individual nurses have not caught up with these professional goals and aspirations. Although many nurses express professionalism on a conscious level, many of their actions show that on a subconscious level they have not made the transition from dependent, caring, female helpers to independent, thinking professionals. Nursing administrators and practitioners must meet the challenge and make this transition in their thinking. Then, their performance, status, and professional position in the health care industry can also change.

SUMMARY

In this chapter, the principles of three self-image models were outlined and applied to the thoughts, beliefs, actions, performance, and achievements of nurses and of the nursing profession.

The personal experiences, environment, and reference groups of nurses have strongly influenced their thoughts and beliefs about their capabilities. Historically, the great majority of nurses have been women, and women have been socialized to be more dependent on other people, to focus on external sources of power rather than on themselves, and to avoid risky situations.

A person's thoughts and beliefs determine that person's self-image. Historically, nurses have been socialized to have the self-image of giving, caring, and dedicated helpers who need to follow directions, to be respectful, and never to make mistakes.

A person's behavior, actions, and performance are consistent with that person's self-image. The actions of many nurses show that they have compromised self-images and comparatively low levels of self-esteem when compared with other professionals. Many nurses desire professional status but have not yet internalized the self-image of a professional and assumed total responsibility for their lives.

The following chapters will describe detailed plans of action for nurses to implement in various professional roles in order to develop and enhance their professional self-images and improve their performance and achievements.

Display 2-1
SOCIALIZATION FACTORS
AFFECTING NURSES

Experiences

1. Nursing school has taught nurses never to make mistakes.
2. Nurses have been taught to help others.
3. Nurses are taught that they must always respect physicians and superiors.
4. Nurses are taught that they are responsible for their patients' health.
5. Nurses are taught that they need to be the patient's advocate.
6. Society has taught women that men are superior in leadership and quantitative abilities.
7. Society has taught women that they will make less money than their male counterparts.
8. Society has taught women that they make good nurses, teachers, secretaries, and mothers.
9. Society has taught women that they have the major responsibility for child rearing.

Reference Groups

1. The family has taught women to take care of others and not to complain.
2. Mothers and fathers have taught women not to get angry and to "always be good."
3. Men have taught women that they are not good with numbers or dealing with difficult business situations.
4. Men have taught women that they are more emotional.
5. Physicians have taught nurses that they are to respond to physicians' needs and that they are not as smart as physicians.
6. Nursing faculty have taught nursing students to follow directions and never to question authority figures.
7. Women have taught other women not to trust one another.

Display 2-1 *(continued)*
**SOCIALIZATION FACTORS
AFFECTING NURSES**

8. Men have taught women that they need to perform twice as well as men to compete with them.
9. Men and women have taught women that housework is their major responsibility.

Heredity

1. Heredity determines only whether a person is a male or female.

Environment

1. The family determines which members get educational support for their careers.
2. The time period in which a person grows up determines what careers society sanctions for each gender.
3. The economic and health care environment determines who goes into the profession of nursing based on economic support, societal pressures, economic situation of family, etc.
4. The geographical environment determines the availability of educational opportunities for various careers.
5. The supply and demand for nurses determines who goes into the profession.

3

Developing a Professional Self-Image for the Student and the Clinical Nurse

This chapter defines and applies some concepts relevant to the development of a positive self-image for the student and the new clinical nurse. It presents a concrete plan of action for the new clinical nurse to develop a professional self-image and to enhance performance and achievements. In addition, it outlines the effects of a positive professional self-image on individual nurses, patients, the organization, and the profession.

SOCIALIZATION OF THE STUDENT OR NEW CLINICAL NURSE

A study of the history of nursing reveals a strong religious orientation from the time of Florence Nightingale up to the 1950s. The early mission of the profession, as today, was to provide health care services to humankind. Early nursing leaders felt that the people who provided these services needed to have a strong socialization in ethics and self-discipline because they would care for and be responsible for people who were physically or emotionally compromised.

Initially, nurses were trained in hospitals and learned by observing and working with experienced nurses. Student nurses lived in dormitories near or connected to the hospital, and much of their professional socialization came through strict rules and expectations that

KEY CHAPTER CONCEPTS

Key Concept #1

Your professional self-image is determined by the thoughts you think on an ongoing basis.

Key Concept #2

Your professional self-image determines your performance and achievements.

Key Concept #3

You can program your mind and body to accomplish any goal you desire by writing the goal down, verbalizing the goal through positive affirmations, and visualizing the goal through pictures and daydreaming techniques.

Key Concept #4

You have the mental, emotional, and physical capability to accomplish any idea or concept that enters your conscious mind.

Key Concept #5

A goal is a measurable, concrete objective that is written down and mentally committed to. A wish is a vague objective that you would like to reach but that you do not write down or make a commitment to accomplish.

Key Concept #6

An affirmation is a positive, declarative statement that, when repeated in a consistent and ongoing manner, influences what your brain believes to be true about yourself.

Key Concept #7

Whether you think you can accomplish something or think you cannot accomplish something, what you think will always be right.

governed their behavior twenty-four hours a day. Values such as hard work, self-discipline, respect for authority, and following established rules and regulations were incorporated into the daily schedule and life of student nurses. People who could not cope with long work and study hours, difficult patients, demanding assignments, and demanding physicians and supervisors were dropped from the program or left on their own accord.

Students usually carried full patient assignments within nine months of entering their nursing education and were expected to care for patients and conditions they may have had minimal instruction or training in. Nursing faculty and supervisors had high expectations of their students. Tough-minded students survived; those who were overwhelmed or noncompliant dropped out.

Over the past twenty years, nursing education has moved into community college and university settings. Some students live in dormitories on college campuses; many others live with parents or in their own apartments. In the late 1980s, a higher percentage of older students began entering nursing as a second career or as a first career after their children were grown or after a divorce. Some students live with their husbands and families or, in the case of single women, with their children. In these educational settings, students take more liberal arts courses and receive less clinical nursing experience when compared with hospital-based diploma programs. For example, their clinical nursing experiences may include only observing surgical procedures rather than learning how to scrub and circulate for those procedures. In almost all nursing education programs, student nurse clinical assignments do not resemble actual patient care assignments for a practicing professional nurse. Current clinical nursing education rarely provides the actual experience of being a practicing professional nurse in a real hospital setting.

One strength of the hospital-based diploma program was that nursing students actually experienced the roles, responsibilities, and pressures of professional practice throughout their education. If they did not like the roles and responsibilities of the professional nurse, they could drop out of the program to seek other career opportunities. Today, many new clinical nurses experience what the literature calls "reality shock" when they begin practicing after graduating from a two- or four-year nursing program. This shock occurs because the roles, responsibilities, and pressures of the practicing nurse are quite different from those experienced by the student.

BELIEFS, SELF-IMAGE, AND PERFORMANCE

The challenge for nursing today is to develop the professional self-image of the new graduate that has had minimal clinical experience in a very challenging clinical career. Minimal experience in clinical nursing usually results in a significant level of insecurity in the new graduate nurse. On top of this insecurity about their clinical skills, many new nurses have grown up with negative programming in which their weaknesses seem to have received more attention than their strengths. These factors often result in a compromised professional self-image. Professional self-image determines performance and achievements *(Key Concept #2)*. By taking action to develop a strong, positive professional self-image, new nurses can dramatically enhance their professional performance, achievements, and the quality of patient care they provide.

Key Concept #1 states that your professional self-image is determined by the thoughts you think on an ongoing basis. This concept was first recorded in the Bible in the passage, "As a man thinketh, so is he." Approximately 85% of a person's success or failure is related to that person's thoughts or attitude, while only 15% is based on aptitude. Despite the numerous self-help books and tapes available on the market, many people still have negative attitudes that limit their personal and professional success.

People who have positive self-images are positive thinkers or optimists. People who have poor self-images are usually negative thinkers or pessimists. Today, the concept of positive thinking is at the forefront of many fields of knowledge and is no longer considered superstition. By increasing the number of nurses that are optimists and positive thinkers, our profession can enjoy a significantly brighter and successful future.

Martin Sigelman, a noted psychologist at the University of Pennsylvania, reported that optimists are more successful than their equally talented and competent pessimistic colleagues in business, education, sports, and politics (cited in Olsen, 1988). Sigelman studied the way people explain the disappointments in their life. He found that optimists perform better than their pessimistic counterparts because they are persistent, take more risks, and try new things because they expect positive outcomes. Optimists expect to encounter obstacles but believe that they can overcome them. Pessimists, on the other hand, are more cautious because they expect poor outcomes. When faced with an obstacle, pessimists view the obstacle as a failure and quit because they have little confidence in their own abilities to overcome it. Persistence has been described as a measure of self-confidence and is a key attribute of success.

DEVELOPING A PROFESSIONAL SELF-IMAGE

Setting Goals

Only 5% of the population actually sets specific, written-down goals (Tracy, 1986). Usually, people have difficulty setting and following through with goals for two major reasons: because they fear failure and because they never really learned how to set goals. Setting a goal involves a risk because there is always the chance that you will not accomplish it. Some people never learned how to set goals because their role models (parents and teachers) never set goals. Most people go through grade school and high school without receiving even one hour of instruction on how to set goals.

Some people also have difficulty following through with a goal-setting plan because it appears so deceptively simple. Goal-setting is simple to implement but requires a significant amount of self-discipline to maintain. Self-discipline is a key factor that separates winners from losers. It is fairly easy for people to make a resolution to change their lifestyle and habits when they experience a significant emotional or physical event that results in suffering and pain. However, it is more difficult to follow up with a resolution after the initial pain passes. For example, when people feel good physically, they generally see no reason to eat properly, stop smoking, drink in moderation, or exercise. However, when they experience a significant physical or emotional event such as a heart attack or stroke, they become very motivated to alter their behavior and lifestyle and to follow a recommended medical regimen to improve their health. After they begin to feel better, however, they have a tendency to return to their former lifestyle and habits. This is why many people fail to follow through with New Year's resolutions or self-improvement plans. People usually have to feel pretty bad about themselves or be quite depressed before they seek professional help or read books or articles in order to enhance their lives. People usually do not take action on an issue much before they really have to.

Despite this characteristic of human nature, you can program your mind and body to accomplish any goal you desire by writing the goal down, verbalizing the goal through positive affirmations, and visualizing the goal through pictures and daydreaming techniques (Key Concept #3). This plan provides you with an option to enhance the quality of your personal and professional life before you experience significant discomfort or frustration.

Many people set goals by thinking about what they want to avoid rather than what they want to accomplish. For example, people spend a lot of time thinking about not having enough money, not getting sick, or not getting the right breaks or enough recognition in life. They often fail to focus specifically on what they actually want or desire to actualize in their lives. The problem with this kind of thinking is that the brain, because of its cybernetic properties which direct it to specific goals, cannot actualize a negative or avoidance situation. It can only actualize the specific things that the mind thinks about most of the time.

The only way to change the direction of your life is by changing the direction of your dominant thoughts. By changing the nature and direction of your dominant thoughts, your brain can change the direction of your life. Your expectations determine your outcomes as well as the outcomes you expect from others. If you expect positive outcomes for your life, your brain will direct you to do what needs to be done to attain those positive expectations. Winners manufacture expectations of positive outcomes for themselves that in turn result in positive outcomes. They adopt an attitude that they have the ability to make positive outcomes happen for themselves, rather than adopting the position that their external environment chooses the outcomes that come to them. This manufacturing of positive expectations always results in a renewed sense of energy, enthusiasm, and self-confidence, all of which contribute to faster realization of positive outcomes.

Positive manufactured expectations are driven by your belief system about the world and your place in the world. Your beliefs are a product of your self-image or the dominant thoughts you hold about yourself. You can control the dominant thoughts you have of yourself, thereby controlling the positive outcomes that you expect will come to you.

PROFESSIONAL SELF-IMAGE
DEVELOPMENT PLAN

This section presents a very specific plan of action that can help the student or new clinical nurse develop a positive and professional self-image. Following the simple steps in this plan can dramatically enhance thoughts, actions, performance, achievements, and overall quality of life, and can allow the new nurse to embark on a very productive and successful career. The plan involves setting and writing down specific professional goals and short-term objectives, and developing affirmations and visualizations to actualize these goals.

Step One:
Assume Total Responsibility for Yourself

The first step to professional development is to make the decision to take total responsibility and accept accountability for your personal life and your professional life. This decision frequently follows an extended episode of disillusionment about your life. The decision includes making the commitment to identify and accomplish the personal and professional goals that you strongly desire to attain. It also includes refusing to blame anyone or anything for what has happened to you in the past or present, or will happen in the future.

An affirmation is a positive, declarative statement that when repeated in a consistent and ongoing manner influences what your brain believes to be true for you *(Key Concept #6).* The following list of sample affirmations may assist you in internalizing the concept that you are totally responsible and accountable for where you are in your life. Positive affirmations will be discussed in greater detail later in the chapter.

1. I am totally responsible for my life.
2. If it is going to be, it is up to me.
3. I am totally accountable for my professional career.
4. I am totally responsible for my nursing practice.
5. I am totally responsible for my own happiness.
6. I am totally responsible for where I am at all times in my life.

Step Two:
Define a Professional Career Goal

The second step in professional development is to identify a professional goal that you strongly desire to accomplish in the next two years. When setting professional goals, you need to identify what you feel you have to accomplish to be a successful professional nurse. This is not what your mother, father, or significant other considers important, but what you feel is important to accomplish as a professional. It is also important to understand that no goal is foolish if you really want it.

A goal has to be something that you really want and have a strong desire to attain. If either of these conditions is not met, you will have difficulty accomplishing the goal. Too many times people fall short of their goals because they never valued the goals in the first place. Remember, you are designing your life. Your goals must be the ones you have a strong desire to attain so that you can overcome the obstacles inherent in all goal attainment.

A goal is a measurable, concrete objective that is written down and mentally committed to *(Key Concept #5)*. Goals must be written down on paper. If you are not willing to invest the time or effort to write a goal down, you do not have a strong desire to accomplish it and you will not be willing to pay the price to attain it.

Wishes, on the other hand, are objectives that you would like to have but you do not commit to. Few people attain their wishes because they do little to accomplish them. You have the capacity to attain all your wishes, however, if you are willing to invest the appropriate time, energy, and effort to convert them into written-down goals. You have the mental, emotional, and physical capability to accomplish any idea or concept that enters your conscious mind *(Key Concept #4)*.

Goals are never accomplished without paying a price. The price you need to pay to attain a professional goal may be the cost and time associated with going back to school to complete a particular degree or develop a specific clinical skill. The price might be giving up some of your free time to network, study, or write. Or it might be having to move and leave familiar surroundings or change spouses or jobs. Casual observers are not always aware of the price a person has to pay to accomplish a significant goal, and often they attribute significant accomplishments to luck or natural ability. However, behind all

---

Display 3-1
SAMPLE PROFESSIONAL GOALS FOR THE
NEW CLINICAL NURSE

By _____ , 19 _____ , I am
a competent, caring clinical nurse.

By _____ , 19 _____ , I am
capable of caring for critically ill patients in the intensive care
setting.

By _____ , 19 _____ , I am
a competent mobile intensive care nurse.

By _____ , 19 _____ , I am
a confident team leader on my unit.

By _____ , 19 _____ , I am
a clinical level three Registered Nurse in my hospital.

By _____ , 19 _____ , I am
a confident, competent public health nurse.

---

luck and natural ability is a hidden price the person had to pay to
accomplish their goals.

Display 3-1 provides a sample list of professional goals for a new
clinical nurse. These professional goals are written as positive statements, in the present tense, with specific deadlines. Goals have to be
worded as positive statements in the present tense. Wording them in
the present tense allows you to program your brain to believe that the
condition already exists, rather than that the condition will exist sometime in the unknown future. Goals must always be worded as positive
statements because the brain cannot accept a goal that attempts to
avoid or prevent something from happening. Deadlines are important

in setting goals because they communicate a sense of urgency and force you to act. Many people tend to procrastinate or put things off. Setting a deadline forces you to take action and counteracts this inclination to procrastinate.

Step Three:
Professional Self-Assessment

The third step in professional development is a professional self-assessment. To accomplish this step, complete the professional self-image assessment in Display 3-2. This assessment form consists of three columns of information. The first column identifies important characteristics that are pertinent for professionals. The third column outlines an ideal self-image for a professional clinical nurse. The middle column is designed for you to complete a self-assessment of your current self-image in relationship to the professional characteristics identified in the first column.

Use short phrases or single words to describe yourself in relation to each of the professional criteria. Then compare your present self-image with the ideal professional self-image traits identified in column three. This activity forces you to assess where you currently are with respect to important characteristics of a professional clinical nurse.

Completing a self-assessment is usually an uncomfortable task because it involves taking a critical look at yourself. However, you need to have a clear and objective assessment of your current status in order to determine what you need to do to attain your desired professional goals. It is difficult to set short-term objectives and priorities for your career if you are not in touch with your current situation.

Some people never perform a self-assessment. This occurs because they feel that they get enough negative feedback from others around them, because it is a painful experience, and because they usually do not understand the importance of the process. Looking at yourself objectively requires a strong, positive self-image, confidence in your ability to improve your shortcomings, and a belief that you are totally responsible for your present and future position in life.

People with poor self-images tend to avoid any and all situations in which they might receive negative feedback. This avoidance pattern results in defensive behavior and an inability to hear constructive

(text continues on page 64)

Display 3-2
PROFESSIONAL SELF-IMAGE ASSESSMENT

Professional Characteristics	Your Current Self-Image	Professional Nurse Image
College Education		Baccalaureate degree
Knowledge Base		Clinical nursing
		Organization theory
		Decision-making
		Problem-solving techniques
		Health care economics
Professional Practice		Clinically competent
		Able to delegate and follow up with nonprofessional staff
		Able to organize and prioritize interventions on behalf of patients and fellow staff
		Able to assume total responsibility for coordination of all care provided to patients assigned to care
		Able to assess, plan, administer, and evaluate clinical care provided by all disciplines to patients
		Able to function as shift leader of a nursing unit

(continued)

Display 3-2 *(continued)*
PROFESSIONAL SELF-IMAGE ASSESSMENT

Professional Characteristics	*Your Current Self-Image*	*Professional Nurse Image*
		Able to function as expert nursing resource for other professionals
		Willing and able to assume responsibility and accountability for patient care outcomes
Physical and Personal Appearance		Self-confident
		Neatly groomed
		Attractive uniforms
		Appropriate weight for height
		Healthy appearance
		Good posture
Compensation		Salaried mentality
		Capable of communicating assertively to superiors regarding salary
		Long-term career focus
Professional Contributions		Attends professional meetings
		Member of professional nursing organization
		Makes contributions to nursing department by identifying solutions to departmental problems

Display 3-2 *(continued)*
PROFESSIONAL SELF-IMAGE ASSESSMENT

Professional Characteristics	*Your Current Self-Image*	*Professional Nurse Image*
		Supports colleagues
		Motivated to make a contribution to the profession
Professional Communication		Assertive communications with all stakeholders
		Able to provide peers with direct, constructive feedback on their professional performance
		Complete and comprehensive patient documentation
		Articulates thoughts and ideas well verbally and in writing
		Does not blame others or make excuses for poor patient outcomes or processes
		Does not exhibit defensive behavior
Self-Control		Able to maintain control over emotions in public

suggestions that are designed to help them be more successful in their professional lives. Once people internalize total responsibility for their lives and happiness and learn how to receive constructive feedback in a supportive environment, it becomes much easier for them to receive feedback without becoming defensive. Defensive behavior is not consistent with professional behavior. People in the nursing profession must overcome this behavior so that the profession can take a leadership position in the health care industry.

The peer review process is an example of a formal way to receive constructive feedback on professional performance. When first engaged in, peer review can be a very threatening experience. Many organized medical staffs are finding it difficult to implement the mandatory peer review process outlined by the Joint Commission on Accreditation of Healthcare Organizations. It has been very difficult for some physicians to give and receive feedback on their professional practices. Peer review is threatening because many people have compromised self-images and lack experience in the process.

After developing a strong, positive self-image, a person becomes more willing to receive constructive feedback. In fact, according to some contemporary writers (Tracy, 1986; Kanter, 1977, 1988; Garfield, 1986), high performers constantly go out of their way to get feedback on their performance so that they can continually exceed their past performances.

Nursing peer review should be implemented to improve nurses' ability to provide and accept constructive feedback and to reduce defensive behavior. After becoming comfortable with the process, nurses can seek out feedback from their peers to improve their future performances without feeling threatened. This process can have a strong, positive impact on the self-images of clinical nurses and can strengthen their working relationships with one another. As a result of this feedback process, the practice of nursing can be enhanced. Enhanced nursing practice will improve patient care and organizational outcomes.

Step Four:
Develop Short-Term
Professional Objectives

After completing your professional self-assessment, develop some six- to twelve-month professional objectives that will help you move toward

---

Display 3-3
SAMPLE SHORT-TERM OBJECTIVES

Short-Term Objectives   *Date Accomplished*

---

1. Enroll in a graduate program   _____

2. Complete an assertiveness training program   _____

3. Attain the Registered Nurse 4 level in my hospital   _____

4. Receive an above satisfaction performance rating   _____

5. Complete mobile intensive care nurse training   _____

6. Complete a critical care course   _____

---

your desired two-year professional goal. To develop these objectives, refer to your professional self-assessment and pick three or four criteria for which your current self-image varies significantly from the ideal professional self-image. Develop short-term objectives that will move you closer to your desired professional goal over the next year. For example, if your competence in relating to physicians in an assertive manner is not where it needs to be, you could develop a short-term objective such as: *By _____ , 19____ , my interpersonal communications with physicians is assertive and effective.*

These short-term objectives can be written in your diary or calendar so that you can easily refer to them throughout the year. You can also include a column to document the date you actually accomplished each objective. At the end of the year, this documentation can provide you with gratification for the goals you accomplished. Display 3-3 provides a sample list of short-term objectives to assist you in moving closer to your long-term professional career goals.

Step Five:
Program the Servomechanism
in Your Mind

After developing your short-term objectives, focus on programming your mind to accomplish the goals and objectives you have set.

Writing Down Your Goal

The first method of programming is to write down your desired goal and objectives. By writing your goals and objectives down, you are programming them into your brain just like you enter data into a computer.

A second way to program a goal or objective into your brain is to find a picture of your goal or the way you will look after you have attained your goal. When your brain sees a picture of exactly what you desire, it will do what needs to be done to accomplish that goal. When you repeatedly look at the picture of exactly what you desire, the servomechanism in your brain receives a very clear picture of the desired outcome and directs your body to do what needs to be done to accomplish the goal. The more clearly you can see the goal in your mind, the sooner the servomechanism in your brain moves you toward it.

Take adequate time to find a picture of exactly what you will look like after you have accomplished your professional goal. Your picture should include the exact way you will be dressed, your ideal weight and professional image, your ideal makeup and hairstyle, and the appropriate accessories for your professional goal.

Physical appearance is a significant component of the complete image of a competent professional nurse. For example, if you wish to become a critical care nurse in two years, you should be familiar with the dress code and professional appearance of critical care nurses in your organization. You should pay close attention to the type of accessories they use in their professional practice, such as stethoscopes, penlights, and other items that are a part of their professional image.

Investigate the availability of critical care courses or internships in your hospital or community. You should understand the prerequisites, abilities, and skills you need to become a critical care nurse so that you can position yourself to acquire these skills and abilities. Identify what you need to know, what you need to look like, with whom you need to network, and when you need to take specific actions to accomplish your goal within your two-year time frame. You need to learn how to look and act the part of being a critical care nurse from the perspective of others in your organization. This can be accomplished by closely observing and emulating the positive critical care role models in your organization.

Positive Affirmations

A third method of programming the servomechanism in your brain is a verbal technique called "positive affirmations." An affirmation is a positive, declarative statement that, when repeated in a consistent and ongoing manner, influences what your brain believes to be true for you *(Key Concept #6).* This verbal programming technique includes the development and repetition of positive affirmations that actualize your professional goals and objectives. Affirmations are positive statements, in the present tense, that articulate a desired situation or condition. They are a verbal and auditory way of programming your brain to bring your desired goals and objectives into reality.

Affirmations are not a new influence to anyone. When a person's inner voice engages in the act of worrying about something, or when the person concentrates on a fear or negative situation, that person is influenced by negative affirmations. Negative affirmations are negative statements that are repeated unconsciously, such as when a person worries about failing a test, performing poorly, or not having enough money to pay the bills. These negative affirmations have a powerful influence on all of us in our daily lives. However, you can turn that powerful negative influence into a powerful positive influence in your life through the use of positive affirmations.

To move toward your desired professional goal, you need to develop positive affirmations for each one of your short-term objectives. There are three simple guidelines to follow when developing positive affirmations.

First, positive affirmations must be developed using positive action words rather than negative words. For example, a positive affirmation to stop smoking should be worded *I feel good about myself as a nonsmoker,* rather than *I will quit smoking.*

The brain only acknowledges action words and positive modifiers when listening to affirmations. It does not accept or acknowledge negative words such as *not, quit, never,* or *don't.* It only acknowledges programmed statements such as "I = nonsmoker" or "I = smoker."

Second, positive affirmations need to be very specific. For example, positive affirmations cannot be statements such as *I will be successful.* Positive affirmations need to have a specific outcome or goal, such as: *I am the clinical nurse 4 on my unit.*

Affirmations must be specific and precise so that you know when and if you actually accomplish them. This specificity requires taking a risk and committing to a very specific role or accomplishment. People tend to avoid this level of specificity because of a fear of failure. They cope with this fear of failing by not setting or committing to any specific goals in the first place. Goal-setting always involves risk and paying a price. However, if you do not set goals, you may be paying a higher price in the form of unhappiness and unfulfillment.

Committing to a specific goal involves a significant level of confidence in your ability to accomplish the goal. This creates anxiety for many people. This anxiety must be overcome for you to be able to experience the increased self-confidence that accompanies goal accomplishment. Once this success has been experienced, you become more willing and able to set higher, riskier goals.

The third guideline for developing positive affirmations is that they need to be worded as if the goal has already been accomplished rather than as if it will occur sometime in the future. This enables you to accomplish the goal in a quicker time frame. For example, if you set a professional goal to become a critical care nurse, your positive affirmation should be worded: *I am a competent critical care nurse.* By using the present tense, you are programming your brain to act as if you already are a competent critical care nurse. When your brain internalizes this affirmation as truth, it will direct you to act, talk, and make decisions and choices as if you were already a critical care nurse.

By reprogramming your self-image as a competent critical care nurse, you will behave in ways that are consistent with being a competent critical care nurse. When nurse managers interview clinical nurses to train as critical care nurses in the organization, they look for nurses that exhibit the traits, actions, and behaviors of potential critical care nurses. By repeating the positive affirmation that you are a competent critical care nurse, you can develop the characteristics and behaviors necessary to be selected for this opportunity.

Develop at least one affirmation for your desired professional goal and for each of your short-term objectives. Display 3-4 (pp. 70–71) provides a sample list of positive affirmations for professional career goals and short-term objectives.

To program your self-image to accomplish your desired professional goal, repeat each of your affirmations ten times in the morning and ten times in the evening for two weeks. The following strategies will help you to follow through with your positive affirmations:

1. Write your affirmations on an index card and tape them to your bathroom mirror. This will serve as a reminder to say them ten times out loud when you are getting ready for work in the morning and getting ready for bed in the evening.
2. Tape record yourself saying your positive affirmations and listen to the tape on your way to and from work.
3. When you are in a boring meeting, getting your hair or nails done, or waiting in the dentist's or doctor's office, write your affirmations down on paper. This allows you to turn all your unproductive waiting time into productive time that will help you to accomplish your goals faster.
4. Promise yourself a specific reward if you follow through with repeating your affirmations for two weeks. Your reward can be a shopping spree, a special night out, or a new outfit. Be sure that the reward you select is a strong personal motivator. It is best if the reward involves a financial incentive of some type because people tend to follow through more consistently when money is on the line.

Visualization

Visualization is a fourth technique for reprogramming your brain to actualize your desired professional goal. Visualization is the process of daydreaming or creating a movie in your mind of the specific situation, condition, or goal that you desire. Seeing your desired goal or scenario in your mind in every detail will cause the servomechanism in your brain to direct your body to act to accomplish your desired picture.

Visualization is the process that most relaxation and biofeedback techniques are based on. It relies on the fact that your mind cannot differentiate between what is real and what is vividly imagined. If you

(text continues on page 72)

Display 3-4
SAMPLE PROFESSIONAL GOALS AND
POSITIVE AFFIRMATIONS

*Professional Goals and
Short-Term Objectives*

Positive Affirmations

1. By _____ , 19 _____ ,
I am enrolled in a Master's
program that will enhance
my career.

I am a competent graduate
student.

I can do anything I set my
mind to.

I am challenged by my graduate
studies.

2. By _____ , 19 _____ ,
I have mastered my assertive
communication skills to be
more effective with
physicians, peers, and
superiors.

I feel good about my assertive
communication skills with all my
colleagues.

Physicians respect my clinical
judgment.

I always take responsibility for
communicating directly and
empathetically with all my
contacts.

Physicians respect me as a
professional nurse.

3. By _____ , 19 _____ ,
I am a competent and
confident clinical practitioner.

I am a confident and caring
nurse.

I am a great nurse.

I am constantly learning new
things from my peers,
physicians, and patients.

Display 3-4 *(continued)*
SAMPLE PROFESSIONAL GOALS AND
POSITIVE AFFIRMATIONS

Professional Goals and Short-Term Objectives	*Positive Affirmations*
	I am a valuable asset to my unit and organization.
	I am a great professional role model for nursing.
	I am totally responsible for my professional practice.
	I am well respected by my peers and superiors for my excellent nursing care.
	I feel good about my clinical skills.
	My patients respond positively to my nursing care.
4. By _____ , 19 _____ , I have completed a critical care course.	I feel good about my critical care nursing skills. I am a competent critical care nurse.
5. By _____ , 19 _____ , I have completed a mobile intensive care nurse (MICN) training program.	I am a competent and skillful MICN. I love my role as a MICN. I make a valuable contribution as a MICN.

imagine or visualize a scenario long enough, you will begin to believe that it is true, and your body will act in ways consistent with that belief.

For example, you may have had a painful or unhappy experience that, every time you told the story to someone, you altered slightly to more accurately reflect what you really wanted to happen. Over time, you may have told the altered version so many times that you actually believed your revised version was true and could not remember the real version.

Visualization is a skill being mastered and used increasingly in many different fields. For example, many athletes use visualization to mentally see and rehearse perfect performances before they participate in athletic competitions. By practicing in your mind, you can practice performing perfectly because you control all the variables. Over time, this perfect practice initiated in your mind communicates to your muscles what they need to do automatically to duplicate a perfect performance.

Doe Yamashiro, a leading United States gymnast, visualized herself performing flawlessly as part of her routine Olympic training (Olsen, 1988). She is just one of a growing number of athletes and coaches who believe that the power of visualization is at least as important as physical training in performing well.

In your development as a professional, visualization is an effective tool in assisting you to attain your professional career goals. It allows you to see yourself performing perfectly in your desired professional role. By practicing the appropriate behaviors, skills, and actions for your desired professional role repeatedly in your mind, and by seeing yourself perform perfectly in the role, you prepare yourself to perform perfectly in your desired role. This technique can be used to develop your speaking ability, request raises, sell your ideas to your superior, enhance your athletic abilities, or develop your assertiveness.

The most productive and effective action you can take to accomplish any goal is to be able to see the goal clearly in your mind through programming techniques. You can only actualize or accomplish things you can see in your mind's eye. If you desire a raise, promotion, or competency in some area but your mind sees you being rejected or being a failure, that is exactly what you will actualize. However, if you can visualize yourself as already having accomplished a goal, the hardest part of attaining the goal has been overcome.

The Visualization Process

There are three steps in the visualization process. The first step is to decide what goal or dream you are going to visualize. You may be working on a number of goals in your personal and professional life; however, you can only visualize one at a time.

The second step is to get into a relaxed state. Visualization can make a greater impact on your subconscious mind if you are relaxed. To get into a relaxed state, sit in a comfortable chair with both feet on the ground and your hands in your lap with palms up. Close your eyes and take five deep breaths, inhaling through the nose and exhaling through pursed lips. If you cannot assume this position but have time to daydream, get comfortable, and take five deep breaths.

The third step is to see a picture of your goal in your mind as vividly as possible. Include all the details of your goal and make them exactly the way you want them to be. Your visualization should be in color and should include the sounds, smells, and feelings associated with your desired goal. Include the exact words you would say and the specific actions you would take after attaining your desired professional goal. Include specific things other people in your professional setting are saying and doing.

Repeat this visualization process at least once a day. Each time you visualize, improve on the specific details until it is exactly the way you want it to happen in real life. If your desired goal includes some kind of clinical competence, see yourself executing each action in the technical skill perfectly.

Your muscles will remember what they need to do to duplicate a perfect performance just as if you had physically practiced a skill. The only difference is that visualization can result in perfect practice because you control the variables. Physical practice includes making mistakes and errors that may in turn result in a flawed performance. Combining visualization practice and physical practice is the most effective method of reaching your goal.

Visualizing Professional Career Goals

When visualizing your desired professional goal, create a picture of exactly how you want your life to be after you have accomplished your professional goal. See exactly how you are dressed, what you are doing, what you are saying, and who you are talking to. See the kind of department or area and hospital or organization you are employed in. See yourself performing the actual tasks you would perform in your desired professional role and executing each task perfectly. See yourself interacting positively and effectively with physicians and having them respect your clinical judgment and assessments. Visualize them asking for your advice and relating to you in a collaborative manner. See your peers coming to you for advice and consultation and admiring your professionalism and judgment.

See your patients respond positively and gratefully to your professional and caring bedside manner. See them communicate that you have made a significant impact on their recovery and their life in general. See them make the decision to take personal responsibility for their health status as a result of your influence and patient education efforts.

See yourself interacting assertively and positively with your boss. Visualize yourself receiving a compensation package that reinforces your positive contribution to patient care, your unit, and your organization. See yourself receiving your check and feeling good about being adequately compensated for the excellent job you do. Visualize the exact amount of your compensation, which represents the professional role you fulfill. See yourself going home after work with a feeling of accomplishment, pride, and satisfaction with your nursing contributions.

PROFESSIONAL APPEARANCE

Professional appearance is a key component of actualizing your professional role. Many nurses believe that appearance is a superficial aspect of professionalism. However, your appearance significantly affects how you act and how others respond to you. Professional appearance is made up of physical height and weight, clothes, grooming, makeup, posture, mannerisms, attitude, and verbal and nonverbal communication. Physical appearance is directly related to self-image and drastically affects a person's professional actions and performance. This is especially true in the health care industry because nurses are expected to be healthy role models for their patients, community, and fellow professionals.

A first step in evaluating your physical appearance starts with identifying the ideal weight for your height and body frame. This can be obtained from the American College of Cardiology Table. If you are more than twenty pounds overweight by this standard, you should set a goal to reach your ideal weight. Weight is very important in conveying a healthy and professional physical appearance as a health care professional. People that are more than twenty pounds overweight sometimes have a compromised self-image that needs to be enhanced in order to maximize their professional performance.

Hundreds of books have been written about weight, diets, and the psychological problems associated with weight. Over the past five to ten years, these issues have extended to the subject of eating disorders discussed in the first chapter. Despite the preoccupation our society has with being thin, many nurses experience real health and image problems when they are twenty or more pounds overweight.

If you come to the conclusion that you need to lose weight, locate a picture of someone who is similar to you in height and body frame and is your ideal weight. Cut your head out of a similar-sized picture and paste it over the head of the person in the picture. Put this picture on your refrigerator, bathroom mirror, daily calendar, or car dashboard to reprogram your brain visually to internalize your desired physical appearance. You can only reach your desired or ideal weight if your mind can actually see you at that weight and believes that it is possible.

The first few times you look at this picture, your brain may stimulate you to laugh disbelievingly or make jokes. Later, you will stop laughing, and it is then you will know that your brain is beginning to internalize your weight goal as a possibility.

Take care to select the exact picture that portrays the professional appearance and image that communicates how you want to look. This is very important because you will actualize your picture in every detail. Once your brain starts to believe your goal is possible, you will begin making decisions on subconscious and conscious levels that actualize your goal in every detail.

It may take you anywhere from several days to several months to find the right picture of your ideal professional or physical image. However, set a deadline of no longer than three months to find the picture. If you do not set a deadline, you may procrastinate, lose interest, and return to an old pattern of wishing for things rather than setting specific goals.

In most families, the support of significant others is required to accomplish any significant goal. By putting the picture of your desired goal in a prominent place, such as on your refrigerator, you are also programming your significant others to believe that attaining the goal is possible. They may laugh when you initially put your goal up. However, do not get discouraged. Just wait until they stop laughing; soon after that you will have their support in attaining your goals.

In addition to using this visualization technique, develop three ideal professional appearance affirmations and follow the same procedure for repeating each affirmation ten times twice a day. Sample affirmations to enhance your physical or professional body image appear in Display 3-5.

In addition to visualizing through pictures and reprogramming yourself through positive affirmations, there are a number of other strategies that can help to enhance your physical or professional image. For example, you can purchase a subliminal weight-control tape and listen to the tape at least once a day for two weeks. You can listen almost anywhere, for example, while traveling in your car or in a plane, getting your hair done, and before bed. Subliminal tapes have positive affirmations that can only be heard by your subconscious mind recorded behind ocean waves or music. Listening to subliminal tapes allows positive affirmations to be programmed directly into your subconscious mind while you are engaged in other activities. They bypass your skeptical conscious mind, which often creates roadblocks to the attainment of your goals. As a result of listening to subliminal weight-control tapes, your conscious mind makes different choices regarding your food consumption that can allow you to reduce your intake of unhealthy foods and calories. Subliminal tapes are available in bookstores and through adult education catalogs such as Career-Track and Nightingale Conant. They also include subjects such as goal-setting, image-building, self-determination, health, fitness, self-esteem, time management, and happiness.

If you need to lose weight, it is helpful to identify the specific number of pounds you need to lose and then to set a realistic deadline for losing the weight. Break down the total pounds you need to lose into realistic weekly weight goals. Reward yourself at the end of each week when you reach your weekly weight goal. Foods such as ice cream and cake have been a traditional reward in so many settings, so you will need to identify a number of nonedible rewards that will motivate you. Those rewards could include new clothes, jewelry, a massage, getting a maid, a pedicure, a facial, or getting your hair done

Display 3-5
POSITIVE AFFIRMATIONS FOR PHYSICAL
OR PROFESSIONAL BODY IMAGE

1. I love my slim, healthy body.

2. I am active, attractive, and in demand.

3. I eat only when my body is hungry, not when my mind is hungry.

4. I enjoy socializing with friends without overeating.

5. I like myself with my attractive figure.

6. I deserve to be _____ pounds.

7. It is easy for me to maintain my ideal weight of _____ pounds.

8. I am a healthy role model for my patients, peers, and family.

9. I am proud of my well-groomed professional appearance.

10. My professional appearance communicates my competence as a professional nurse.

11. My healthy professional appearance communicates my confidence in myself.

12. I always role model a healthy lifestyle and appearance.

on a weekly basis. The reward should be something you consider slightly extravagant and out of the ordinary, as well as something that you really value, so that you follow through on your goals.

Another helpful method is to find an outfit that you really like and buy it in the size you will be after you have attained your desired weight goal. Hang the outfit in a very prominent place in your closet or bedroom where you will see it on a daily basis. When you pass the outfit, visualize yourself in it and visualize others admiring you in it. This visualization technique will assist you to get to your goal faster.

No matter how you feel physically or emotionally on any given day, always dress and groom yourself as if you will work with or bump into the person in your organization who can ultimately help you get to your desired professional goal. This strategy accomplishes two things. First, it forces you consistently to look the part of a professionally competent nurse who is working toward a specific career goal. Second, by consistently looking the part, you communicate a professional image to your patients, peers, and superiors. If you consistently look the part, you will consistently act the part of a competent professional. If you do not accept this logic, just think about how you act when you get dressed up versus how you act when you put on a t-shirt and jeans to relax. Dress and appearance really do affect the way you act. Similarly, appearance, dress, and grooming affect how others respond to you. If you consistently wear well-kept-up white uniforms and conservative makeup and are well groomed, patients, physicians, and peers will respond more positively to you than if you wear unkempt uniforms and are not well groomed.

Your professional appearance is also affected by how you walk and carry yourself. Practice standing erect with your head held high and walking with a purpose. While you are engaged in this activity, say to yourself with confidence and feeling: *I'm a great nurse.* You will notice that this exercise instantly makes you feel good about yourself and provides added self-confidence. You can perform this exercise when you prepare for a difficult situation such as a code blue. By walking confidently and erect and saying to yourself "I'm a great nurse" as you get the crash cart, you can rid yourself of the insecurities and fears you may feel in this stressful situation. You will perform better because of this added self-confidence. Using this strategy will allow you to develop over time a bounce in your step and a meaning in your walk. It will provide you with a definite presence when you enter a room, department, or new situation. This professional presence will allow you to stand out in a crowd and will enhance your professional career accomplishments.

STRATEGIES FOR SUCCESS

There are a number of other specific actions that can help you to develop your professional self-image and enhance your performance. For example, you can start a "box of wins." Get a shoebox and start saving all the positive letters, memos, and evaluations you receive from patients, peers, bosses, friends, and physicians that document that you are doing a good job. Save any projects or articles you have written and rewards you have received. When you go through a difficult period in your career or personal life that causes you to get somewhat depressed, go through your box of wins and relive your successes and the feelings that accompanied those successes. This exercise will allow you to get yourself out of your depression and back on a positive track.

Another strategy is to purchase a packet of colored round stickers. Write your positive affirmations on the stickers and put them in key places, such as your car dashboard, notebook, calendar, clock, checkbook cover, or purse, to keep reminding yourself of your goal.

When you get frustrated or start to feel sorry for yourself, make a list of twenty things that you are grateful for. Your depression will soon leave because you will see that the positive things in your life far outweigh the negative things. This exercise forces you to look for the good and positive things in your life rather than dwell on the negative things and feel sorry for yourself.

Constantly be on the lookout for motivational tapes and positive experiences and influences to counteract the negative programming. People are constantly being bombarded by negative stories, experiences, and people in the newspaper, on television, and at work. These influences negatively program them unconsciously to expect the worst. You need to read, listen, and surround yourself with an equal amount of positive messages, people, and expectations to counteract these negative influences. Human beings are social creatures and are strongly affected by the positive or negative influences that surround them.

Avoid negative people at all costs because their negativity is very contagious. You cannot afford to have someone else's poor self-image and skepticism rub off on you and convince you that you cannot accomplish your goals or that the odds are against you. Make a conscious effort to associate with people who have a positive outlook on life and who you feel are winners. You will emulate their attitudes and actions on a unconscious level. The impact of your immediate reference group has a significant influence on your own attitudes and beliefs. A positive, winning attitude is contagious. When you associate with positive, winning people, you will begin seeing things the way they do. You will find yourself talking about how to actualize positive outcomes, and you will receive the encouragement and optimism you need to accomplish your goals. Winners will tell you that you can do anything you set your mind to. If you associate with these people long enough, you will begin to believe them.

Identify a positive, experienced, competent clinical nurse in your organization whom you admire. Watch how that nurse acts, looks, behaves, and communicates with physicians, administrators, peers, and superiors. Imitate his or her actions and behaviors in order to learn how to act more professionally. Ask this nurse to assist you in your own professional growth and development by providing you with constructive feedback on your clinical and professional appearance and performance.

RESULTS OF PROFESSIONAL DEVELOPMENT

The results of implementing a professional development plan can be dramatic. You can accomplish every goal you set out to attain, from specific jobs and skills to new houses and cars.

The effect of nurses developing their professional self-images has potentially dramatic implications for the profession. When nurses enhance their self-images as competent professionals, they are capable of making a significant impact on the nursing profession. That impact includes taking full responsibility for their own nursing practice without blaming others or making excuses for poor patient care processes or outcomes. Being totally accountable for their professional practice results in improved patient care outcomes and an increase in the number of professional role models in the profession.

Increasing the number of professional role models in nursing will attract more people to the profession. This will help alleviate some of the problems associated with the perceived nursing shortage. Taking total accountability for professional practice can also decrease the movement of nurses from facility to facility and job to job, because they do not project their frustrations onto others or the organization. Instead, they work within the framework of their existing role and organization to effect positive changes for themselves, their fellow nurses, and their patients.

SUMMARY

The image of the nursing profession is dependent upon individual professional nurses developing a positive professional self-image. The profession cannot look to external factors to improve or enhance its image. Nurses must look to other nurses who have developed their professional self-images to function as role models for them and then take personal and professional responsibility to develop their own professional self-images.

4

Enhancing the Self-Image of the Experienced Clinical Nurse

This chapter will assist the experienced clinical nurse in evaluating his or her level of satisfaction with career, current role, nursing practice, and organization and in considering the opportunities available to enhance his or her professional satisfaction. It focuses on enhancing the professional self-image of the experienced clinical nurse who may be frustrated or disillusioned with self, career, the profession, the health care organization, or the entire health care system.

It is easy to get in a rut when a person has been performing a specific role or function for an extended period of time or when the person becomes comfortable in a specific role. In many instances, this situation is comfortable but not necessarily satisfying and rewarding. In some instances, the situation is the only option the experienced nurse perceives as viable. This chapter presents some available alternatives and outlines a concrete plan to assist the experienced nurse in enhancing professional satisfaction and sense of fulfillment.

SOCIALIZATION AND ENVIRONMENT OF THE PRACTICING NURSE

As mentioned previously, the environment of health care organizations has historically been security-oriented and has generally attracted security-oriented people. Some believe that professionals in the public

KEY CHAPTER CONCEPTS

Key Concept #1

Your perception of your external environment is directly related to your internal perception of yourself.

Key Concept #2

You have total responsibility for your feelings, actions, and career failure or success.

Key Concept #3

The rewards and recognition of advanced education and skills result from the application of that knowledge.

Key Concept #4

Your level of professional fulfillment and satisfaction is directly related to the contributions you make to the profession.

sector trade the opportunity for high-paying positions in the private sector for the perceived job security of the public sector. This results in a considerable number of experienced nurses remaining in the same clinical specialty and same role for many years. Although these nurses are very knowledgeable in their clinical areas and can perform exceptionally well, this narrow focus can contribute to a familiar routine that can breed contempt, frustration, and burn-out.

If you are one of these nurses, you may feel trapped by your own level of expertise and specialization. You may feel that you have to pay a high price to leave the safety and security of your known specialty to seek new opportunities or challenges. This price usually includes learning new skills and a new body of knowledge, starting at the bottom of the clinical hierarchy in a new specialty, and exposing your vulnerability and lack of experience in another clinical, management, educational, or research setting.

The price and the associated risk of failing in another specialty or role is too great for some nurses. As a result, they continue to function in the area that they are comfortable with, even though they may have a significant level of dissatisfaction with their professional life. Other experienced nurses fear rejection by their co-workers if they leave to seek new learning opportunities and challenges. This fear of rejection can be so great that some nurses remain in their specific clinical specialty, department, or role despite the fact that they do not enjoy their work.

There is nothing wrong with functioning in a certain clinical area for a long period of time. There is no reason to change professional roles if you can maintain the challenge and stimulation you need professionally. However, if you dread going to work, watch the clock constantly while at work, or look for reasons to stay home or to go home early, you need to consider another nursing specialty or role. If you do not enjoy what you are doing professionally, you need to take responsibility for your own happiness and job satisfaction and set new professional goals. On the other hand, if you are challenged by your job but are disenchanted with your department, your organization, or yourself, you can increase your professional satisfaction by enhancing your personal and professional self-image.

According to **Key Concept #1,** your perception of your external environment is directly related to your internal perception of yourself. In other words, if you have a positive internal perception of yourself, you will have a positive perception of the external world. Similarly, if you have a negative self-image, your view of your external environment and the world around you will be negative. For example, you may know people who tend to view everything that happens to them positively, no matter how bad the experiences are. These people tend to have strong, positive self-images, and are not immobilized by negative events. You may also know people who have a negative view of the world and everything that happens to them. Even when positive things happen to these people, they are skeptical and believe that they are probably being "set up" for future disasters. These people usually have a negative self-image that affects the way they view the entire world around them.

Nothing in the world has meaning in itself. People interpret specific events and give them meaning. If a person has a poor or negative self-image, that negativity is projected onto the world and the person perceives most things in a negative manner. If a person has a positive self-image, that positive attitude is projected on the world and the person perceives most things in a positive manner.

Reaction to or perception of the world has little to do with the external world and everything to do with what happens inside of a person. This is why two people can witness the same event yet describe it very differently. Their descriptions differ because the two people have different perceptions of what happened based on their past experiences and who they are. Therefore, it is not what happens to a person that is significant, it is how that person interprets what happens that determines happiness or unhappiness, success or failure.

There are some nurses who just cannot be fulfilled, challenged, or happy staying in the profession. If you are one of these persons who is unable to find a niche or role that is satisfying and rewarding for you, you need to identify what you enjoy doing and develop a career goal that is based on that. You cannot feel good about yourself, perform well, or make a contribution to the profession if you do not enjoy what you are doing. In fact, if you stay in nursing and do not enjoy it, you can actually have a negative impact on your patients, fellow professionals, future nursing professionals, and the profession as a whole because of your frustration and unhappiness.

If you are in this situation, take personal and professional responsibility for yourself and the influence you have on others and leave the profession to pursue a career you can enjoy. Despite the increasing demand for professional nurses, no one really benefits when frustrated, disenchanted nurses remain in the profession.

FOCUSING ON WORDS, ACTIONS, AND IMAGE

If you are satisfied with the profession of nursing but are disenchanted with your environment (department, organization, or role), you can benefit from enhancing your perception of yourself as a successful professional. The following common expectations or assumptions about how successful professionals look, act, talk, walk, and think are important in developing a successful professional image:

1. Experienced professional nurses are confident, self-controlled role models for inexperienced nurses.
2. Experienced professional nurses make independent decisions on behalf of their patients, department, and organization in new or difficult situations.

3. Experienced professional nurses take full responsibility and accountability for the outcomes of their nursing practice and never blame, rationalize, or justify.
4. Experienced professional nurses are internally driven and require little direction and supervision.
5. Experienced professional nurses take responsibility for their ongoing, lifelong learning.
6. Experienced professional nurses look for opportunities to make a contribution to the profession, their departments, and their organizations.
7. Experienced professional nurses function as mentors for inexperienced nurses.

Any plan or strategy to enhance your self-image and professional satisfaction as an experienced nurse should focus on incorporating and developing these traits and characteristics into your professional self-image.

You will need to decide on a future professional goal that will enhance your professional satisfaction. Your options at this point in your career include:

1. Staying in your current clinical specialty and enhancing your professional self-image.
2. Learning a new clinical specialty that challenges your talents.
3. Learning a new role within your existing clinical specialty. For example, if you are currently a direct care provider, you could set a goal to become a clinical specialist or function in a higher clinical level.
4. Deciding to become a nurse manager.

If you desire to focus your energy on becoming a nurse manager, implement the plan outlined in Chapter Five for developing a management self-image. If you enjoy your existing role but are disenchanted with your department or organization, consider the plan outlined in this chapter for enhancing your professional self-image as an experienced clinical nurse. If you desire to change your clinical level or role in your existing specialty, you can use the same plan to develop affirmations and visualizations that accurately reflect your desired clinical role.

Your plan to enhance your professional self-image includes deciding to take total responsibility for your career satisfaction, defining your desired professional goal and image, developing short-term objectives to actualize your professional goal and image, developing and repeating positive affirmations to accomplish your goal, and visualizing yourself as the positive experienced nurse you desire to be.

STEPS TO ENHANCE YOUR PROFESSIONAL IMAGE

Step One:
Take Responsibility for Your Professional Satisfaction

The first step to becoming a positive, enthusiastic, experienced nurse is to assume total responsibility for your professional satisfaction by identifying a professional goal or self-image that can assist you in becoming a positive, enthusiastic, contributing professional. You are the only person who can decide if you should stay in your existing specialty, if you need to enhance your professional self-image, or if you need to take on the additional challenge of learning a new specialty or role. You are the only person who knows what you can be happy doing.

If you are currently unhappy or are not stimulated by your professional role, you have the professional responsibility to define what you really enjoy doing and to take action. No one else can or will make this decision for you.

However, changing organizations or roles is not necessarily the answer to professional dissatisfaction. If you have many negative perceptions, the problem may be the way you feel about yourself. If this is the case, changing organizations or roles will not help because you will take your negative feelings and attitudes with you. The most effective way to change your perception of a negative environment is to change your internal beliefs about yourself by enhancing your self-image.

After enhancing your self-image, you may decide that another organization can provide you with greater challenges or opportunities. Then it may be appropriate to change organizations, departments, or roles. When you leave an organization for new opportunities rather than because you believe that the organization has wronged you, you can leave on a positive note and carry a positive attitude with you to your next position.

When you leave an organization with the attitude that it has strengths and weaknesses and you have strengths and weaknesses, you can be successful in making a change. You need to assume half of the responsibility for any mismatch, problem, or situation that you are involved in. If you blame other people, your boss, or the organization entirely for your problems or unhappiness, you are not being professionally responsible. This attitude can become a way of viewing the world that will follow you wherever you go until you change your thinking.

When you leave an organization with strong negative feelings, your dissatisfaction may lie with you rather than with the organization. When you leave an organization with the attitude that the entire organization is wrong or has treated you unfairly, you will carry those negative feelings to the next organization and may duplicate your dissatisfaction in that position.

You can proceed to Step Two when you can assume total responsibility and accountability for your professional success and have eliminated blame, justification, and rationalization from your vocabulary. You can assess whether or not you have accomplished this step by using Display 4-1. If your thoughts have shifted from those listed in the left-hand column to the ideas in the right-hand column, then you can proceed to the second step.

Remember, your professional success is your responsibility. If you are not enjoying your personal or professional life, it is your issue, not anyone else's. Blaming other people or organizations is irresponsible and will keep you from taking action that could make you happy.

Step Two:
Define Your Desired Professional Goal

Write down a specific professional goal that you want to attain. Your professional goal should be written in the present tense with a specific deadline for its accomplishment.

Define your professional goal as precisely and specifically as possible, including:

Display 4-1
ASSESSING YOUR LEVEL OF
PROFESSIONAL RESPONSIBILITY

Irresponsible Thoughts	*Responsible Professional Thoughts*
1. This organization does not provide any in-service or clinical education; therefore, I cannot advance.	1. I need a greater professional challenge and desire to take a critical care course. When is the next class scheduled?
2. There are no career advancement opportunities in this organization.	2. I need to know what to do to become a clinical nurse 3.
3. All administration cares about is making money. They cut staffing, and patient care is deteriorating.	3. Resources are limited in all industries. My challenge is to do the best I can for my patients given the resources I have at my disposal.
4. Nobody respects nurses.	4. I am an experienced clinical nurse and my patients, physicians, and organization give me the respect I deserve most of the time.
5. My manager will not let me work days. My manager is a problem.	5. I need to work days within the next three months for my family situation. If there is not a position open for me by that time, I need to look for a day position in another department or organization. This is my problem.

1. The clinical specialty you want to become proficient in to attain your desired career goal.
2. The specific clinical role or level you desire.
3. The type of unit or department you want to practice in, for example, university setting, community hospital, or outpatient center.
4. The model of care or delivery system you prefer.
5. The pay scale or salary range you believe is commensurate with the role and responsibility you desire.
6. The general location of the organization or part of the country you want to live in.
7. The specific professional image you wish to actualize.
8. The specific professional attitude or feeling you would like to develop.

Sample professional goals for an experienced clinical nurse are listed in Display 4-2.

Step Three:
Professional Self-Assessment

The next step is to complete a professional self-assessment to determine where you currently are in relation to your desired professional goal. Completion of a self-assessment will help you to develop short-term objectives to move you closer to your desired professional goal. To complete your self-assessment, identify the ideal professional profile for your desired goal by completing the right-hand column of the self-assessment form (Display 4-3, pp. 93–95). Then complete the middle column, or your current professional profile, to assess where you currently are in relation to your desired professional goal. By comparing your current professional profile with your desired professional profile, you can identify the areas you need to work on to move you closer to your desired goal.

Step Four:
Develop Short-Term Objectives

After completing your self-assessment, develop three short-term objectives that can be accomplished within one year that will move you
(text continues on page 95)

Display 4-2
SAMPLE GOALS FOR THE EXPERIENCED
CLINICAL NURSE

1. By _____ , 19 _____ ,
   I am a clinical nurse specialist in the critical care department
   of my hospital.

2. By _____ , 19 _____ ,
   I am a competent mobile intensive care nurse (MICN) in a
   level I trauma center in California.

3. By _____ , 19 _____ ,
   I am a mentor for at least two new clinical nurses in my
   department.

4. By _____ , 19 _____ ,
   I am a clinical nurse 3 in my medical surgical unit.

5. By _____ , 19 _____ ,
   I have presented at least two clinical in-services to my fellow
   nurses.

6. By _____ , 19 _____ ,
   I am functioning as an effective charge nurse in my unit.

7. By _____ , 19 _____ ,
   I am cross-trained to function effectively in the critical care
   unit of my hospital.

Display 4-3
SELF-ASSESSMENT FOR THE
EXPERIENCED CLINICAL NURSE

Criteria	Current Professional Profile	Desired Professional Profile
Education	My current education is:	To attain my desired goal I need this education:
Clinical Expertise	I am clinically competent in these areas:	To attain my desired professional goal I need skills and expertise in these areas:
	1.	1.
	2.	2.
	3.	3.
Organization	I am currently employed in the following organization:	I desire a nursing role in the following organization:
Role	I am currently a:	I desire the professional role of a:
Professional Self-Image	I currently have the self-image of a:	I desire the self-image of a:

(continued)

Display 4-3 *(continued)*
SELF-ASSESSMENT FOR THE
EXPERIENCED CLINICAL NURSE

Criteria	Current Professional Profile	Desired Professional Profile
Physical Appearance	Current weight:	Desired weight:
	Current image/ appearance:	Desired image/ appearance:
	Current physical condition:	Desired physical condition:
	Current dress:	Desired dress:
Professional Contributions	To date, my contributions to the profession include:	I want to make the following contributions to the profession:
	1.	1.
	2.	2.
	3.	3.
Residence	I currently live in:	I want to live in:

Display 4-3 *(continued)*
SELF-ASSESSMENT FOR THE
EXPERIENCED CLINICAL NURSE

Criteria	Current Professional Profile	Desired Professional Profile
Professional Communications	My current communication skills are:	I desire the following communication skills:
	My current expertise in verbal communication is:	I desire the following verbal communication skills:
	My current expertise in written communication is:	I desire the following written communication skills:
	My current expertise in public speaking is:	I desire the following public speaking skills:

closer to your desired professional goal. Display 4-4 provides a list of sample short-term objectives that can be accomplished within one year.

Short-term objectives break down larger professional goals into smaller, realistic objectives. Many people can be overwhelmed by the thought of identifying and accomplishing major career changes. By developing short-term objectives, however, you can gradually move yourself closer to a major professional goal or career change.

A major factor in attaining a professional goal is believing that the goal is possible for you to attain. When you set short-term objectives that will move you closer to your larger professional goals, you are more likely to believe that you can attain those goals.

Display 4-4
SAMPLE SHORT-TERM OBJECTIVES FOR THE EXPERIENCED CLINICAL NURSE

1. By _____ , 19 _____ ,
   I completed an assertiveness training course.

2. By _____ , 19 _____ ,
   I weigh 125 pounds and am physically able to run three miles.

3. By _____ , 19 _____ ,
   I presented one clinical in-service to my colleagues.

4. By _____ , 19 _____ ,
   I am clinically competent in caring for patients on an intra-aortic balloon pump.

5. By _____ , 19 _____ ,
   I am an established mentor for a new clinical nurse on my unit.

6. By _____ , 19 _____ ,
   I have enrolled in a Master's degree program to become a clinical nurse specialist.

7. By _____ , 19 _____ ,
   I have enrolled in a surgery externship program to fulfill my goal of becoming a surgical nurse.

Step Five:
Reprogram Your Self-Image to Your
Desired Professional Image

The next step is to reprogram your self-image to accomplish your desired professional goal by developing and repeating positive affirmations for your goal and short-term objectives, and by visualizing yourself having already attained your goal.

The fastest way to reprogram your self-image is to locate a picture of your desired professional goal. This can be created by finding a picture of someone who fits your desired professional profile and is dressed in the appropriate professional attire for your desired goal, and pasting a similar-sized cut-out of your head on the picture. This picture can then be duplicated and placed in prominent places in your home so that you can visually reprogram your subconscious mind to actualize your desired professional goal.

Next, develop at least one positive affirmation to accomplish each of your short-term objectives. The guidelines for developing positive affirmations were outlined in Chapter Three. Display 4-5 provides a sample list of positive affirmations to accomplish short-term objectives for the experienced clinical nurse.

Write your positive affirmations on index cards and tape them in conspicuous places in your house, car, and office. This will help reprogram your subconscious mind to actualize your desired goal. When you have time during the day, such as when waiting for physicians or dentists or traveling on airplanes, write your positive affirmations down.

Say your positive affirmations out loud at least ten times a day. Good times to do this are early in the morning when you are getting ready for work and in the evening when you are getting ready for bed. By saying your affirmations at these times, you set the tone for the day and program your brain to work on your desired professional goal while you sleep.

RE-ENTERING
THE NURSING PROFESSION

A major challenge facing a number of experienced nurses is the decision to re-enter the active nursing workforce after not practicing for a number of years. These nurses usually have been out of the workforce to raise families, return to school, recover from a major illness, manage a household, or pursue another line of work.

If you are an experienced nurse considering returning to active practice, one strategy for meeting this challenge is to revise your existing self-image of an inactive nurse to the self-image of a competent, working clinical nurse. If you are in this situation, develop a number of positive affirmations that describe you as a competent, active

Display 4-5
SAMPLE POSITIVE AFFIRMATIONS FOR THE
EXPERIENCED CLINICAL NURSE

Short-Term Objectives	*Positive Affirmations*
By _____ , 19 _____ , I am an established mentor for one new clinical nurse.	I am making a positive contribution to nursing by being a mentor.
	I feel good about sharing my nursing expertise by being a mentor.
	I enjoy being a mentor to a new clinical nurse.
By _____ , 19 _____ , I weigh 125 pounds and am physically able to run three miles.	I only eat foods that can maintain my fitness and weight goals.
	I feel good about running three miles three times a week.
	I am an excellent health care role model for my patients and colleagues.
By _____ , 19 _____ , I have enrolled in a surgery training program for registered nurses to fulfill my goal of becoming a surgical nurse.	I enjoy the challenge and excitement of being a surgical nurse.
	I am excited about being a scrub nurse at a trauma hospital.

Display 4-6
SAMPLE POSITIVE AFFIRMATIONS FOR THE NURSE RE-ENTERING THE PROFESSION

1. I feel good about returning to clinical nursing.
2. I have completed a refresher course to return to active nursing practice.
3. I am enthusiastic about returning to the nursing profession.
4. I welcome the opportunity to return to clinical nursing.
5. I have the ability and a strong desire to regain my clinical nursing skills.
6. I am anxious to update my skills and knowledge to return to clinical nursing.
7. I can make a positive impact on my patients' health status.
8. I am confident in my clinical nursing skills.

professional in the area that you were employed in before you left active practice. It is not wise to learn a different clinical specialty at the same time that you are experiencing the trauma of re-entering the workforce and attempting to catch up on the clinical changes that have occurred in your absence. The stress of such a change could stretch you to the point of convincing you not to re-enter nursing.

The first priority is to develop a self-image that is consistent with being a competent, practicing clinical nurse. Develop three to five positive affirmations that can assist you in reactivating or enhancing the professional self-image you had when you were a practicing nurse. Display 4-6 provides a list of sample positive affirmations to help you re-enter the active workforce.

Repeat your positive affirmations ten times a day for at least two weeks to reprogram your self-image to one of a practicing nurse.

The next step is to identify a mentor, a person who is currently practicing in your clinical specialty and who agrees to assist you with your re-entry process. Your mentor can help you to accomplish three important objectives.

First, a mentor can help you to identify the resources and

programs available to you to gain the nursing skills you need to re-enter the active workforce, such as re-entry training programs sponsored by community colleges or hospitals and one-to-one hospital-based preceptor programs. Your mentor may have access to people and organizations that you may not have because of your time away from active nursing professionals.

Second, a mentor can function as a coach, counselor, and cheerleader for you during the re-entry process. You most likely will experience a number of frightening, unfamiliar, and frustrating events. Your mentor can help you put things into perspective and encourage you to continue with your goal.

Third, a mentor can function as a tutor on specific clinical advancements, skills, and technology changes in the delivery of patient care. It is best to select a mentor who is in the same clinical specialty because you are more likely to identify with and understand each other, making the mentor relationship mutually beneficial. When nurses share an interest in the same clinical specialty, they can often assist each other to grow professionally.

CONTRIBUTING TO THE PROFESSION

Some nurses may comment that nursing has never really done anything for them, or that the profession is frustrating and does not provide them with the respect, recognition, and benefits they expect. The profession itself is seen as the cause of their plight and unhappiness. In many instances, these comments hurt the image of the profession because they are made to patients, colleagues, children, and other community members.

If you share these feelings, you have not yet learned the basic principle outlined in *Key Concept #4*: Your level of professional fulfillment and satisfaction is directly related to your specific contributions to the profession. This means that you receive rewards from the profession only when and after you have made a contribution.

The implications of this principle are simple yet significant for the profession of nursing. You only receive gratification and fulfillment from the profession to the degree that you make an active and significant contribution to it. If you make small and inconsistent contributions, you will receive small and inconsistent gratification. On the other hand, if you make consistent and substantial contributions to the profession, you will experience a consistent and significant feeling of career satisfaction and fulfillment.

If you expect only to put in your time as a clinical nurse without doing anything extra, you will be dissatisfied professionally. If you never go out of your way to help new colleagues get comfortable with their professional role, attend professional meetings and seminars at your own expense and on your own time, and take the time to develop new policies, procedures, ideas, or models of care that your department needs, you will never experience any professional satisfaction. If you approach your role and profession with the attitude, "What has the profession ever done for me?" you will never feel good about yourself or what you do.

Professional satisfaction comes only after you take the risk of investing your valuable time, efforts, and energy to do something for your department, organization, or the profession that is over and above what is expected. It is only after you ask yourself what you can do for the profession or how you can make a difference for the profession that you will begin to feel good about what you do and about the profession.

When you make sacrifices without concern for pay or recognition, you will begin to feel like the profession is giving you something valuable in return. The secret is that you must initiate the action and make the first investment. Professional satisfaction and fulfillment come only after you make a contribution and pay the price, not the other way around.

Some people never learn this lesson. They participate in a career or profession for many years waiting to feel fulfilled so that they can decide to make a contribution out of gratitude. These people will always feel cheated because they have the principle backwards. If you are experiencing some of these feelings, you can eliminate them from your professional life by deciding to make a consistent and significant contribution to the nursing profession.

There are a number of specific things you can do to make a contribution to the nursing profession. For example, you can actively participate as a member of professional organizations in your clinical area, such as the Association of Operating Room Nurses (AORN) or the American Association of Critical Care Nurses (AACCN), even if your organization does not pay your membership fee or pay you to attend meetings and conferences. Professional membership is the professional responsibility of the individual professional, not the employer's responsibility.

Volunteer to give a presentation at your professional meetings on something you are an expert on. If you are not currently an expert in something, take responsibility to become one. This is one way you can make a unique contribution to the profession. In addition, you can run for professional office or serve your professional organization as a committee member or chairperson.

Attend professional meetings that are held in the evening even if you have worked during the day. Professionals in other fields realize that they need to work outside of their scheduled hours. This is a professional responsibility, and nurses need to incorporate this idea into their thinking.

You can make contributions to the profession by agreeing to help other nurses. For example, you could offer to be a mentor for an inexperienced colleague or participate in recruitment and educational sessions for future nurses at your local high schools and grade schools. Positive role models who espouse the benefits and rewards of being a nurse are important to combat the declining supply of competent, qualified professional nurses. In addition, you could coordinate a Future Nurses' Club at your local high school to inform students and encourage them to become nurses.

Think of ways that you can assist your department, such as working on special projects at home and without pay that will enhance patient care delivery in your department. Be willing to attend special nursing committee meetings at your facility on your own time to redesign models of care for your department. Request authorization to visit fellow professionals at other hospitals on your own time to learn new ideas for patient care delivery that could be useful to your department.

Nursing journals offer opportunities for making contributions to the profession. Write an article for publication on something that you have become an expert on or something that you have successfully implemented in your department. Write a letter to the editor of a nursing journal you receive and share your perspective on a specific article or current nursing issue. Nursing can only progress if we learn from one another's successes.

Stay current and informed in your clinical specialty by conscientiously reading nursing journals and attending seminars on current issues.

EDUCATION AS A MEANS,
NOT AN END

Some nurses are disillusioned about advancing their professional education because of the perceived lack of rewards and recognition they receive from their organization and the profession. They may feel that they should not go back to school to get a Bachelor's or Master's degree because they will not receive a higher salary from their organization for completing such a program. These expectations have serious implications for the profession because they may discourage higher learning and education. However, in other professions and fields this expectation does not exist. A specific degree allows a person to apply and interview for a particular position. It is not a guarantee that the person will receive a raise or a specific position. The person must convince the interviewer that he or she has the ability to perform in the role or can accomplish a specific challenge. Individual performance and marketing of oneself are the only things that really gain recognition and financial rewards. Advanced education in itself is not financially rewarded. Rather, it is one of the means to accomplish an end or interim goal of a specific role, recognition, or accomplishment.

It has been said that knowledge is power. However, this saying is not complete because power does not automatically come from the possession of knowledge. Power only results from the timely and appropriate use of knowledge, which requires taking action of some kind.

For example, if a nurse acquires the knowledge and skills to be a nurse anesthetist but stays employed in the position of a circulating nurse in an operating room, that nurse will not receive the recognition and rewards of being a nurse anesthetist. Similarly, if a nurse returns to a university and completes a Master's degree in clinical nursing but chooses to continue working in a setting which requires only technical nursing skills, that nurse will not realize the financial rewards and recognition associated with the application of the knowledge learned in the Master's program.

Application of knowledge is the key to realizing the recognition and rewards of higher education. No one is ever compensated for merely possessing knowledge that is not applied. To reduce the disenchantment with higher and ongoing education, nurses must realize that application of knowledge yields rewards and recognition and that advanced and continuing education is an investment in their future career promotability and success, not an end in itself.

The short-term reward for advanced education is completing the educational program and knowing that you completed a goal you set for yourself. The long-term reward of education is the ability to function in advanced roles in the future as a result of gaining the prescribed and needed credentials and skills through formal education and professional experience.

However, as long as nurses view advanced and continuing education as an end in itself that demands rewards, they will remain disenchanted and limit their future success and accomplishments, and the profession will be compromised because of the lack of nurses with advanced education and capabilities.

STRATEGIES FOR DAY-TO-DAY
PROFESSIONAL SATISFACTION

On a day-to-day basis, all professionals experience frustration and disenchantment even if they are in desirable positions that they enjoy for the most part. This section provides strategies that can help you to maintain day-to-day professional satisfaction when you are in a role that you enjoy.

Associate only with positive, enthusiastic professional nurses who display a positive professional image. Your reference groups have a strong and significant impact on your attitudes and beliefs; therefore, you will be negatively affected if you associate with nurses who complain or behave as powerless victims. If you continue to associate with these people, you may soon believe that you cannot attain your professional goals and that the world is not treating you fairly.

Kelley identified five categories of followers in organizations: sheep, yes people, alienated, survivor, and effective followers. He defined followers as those lacking initiative or a sense of responsibility. "Sheep" roll their eyes a lot and are frequently heard saying "It's not my job." "Yes people" are also passive and are very compliant about everything. "Alienated" followers are turned off, burned-out, disillusioned, and always right. They never smile. Kelley's fourth type of follower is the "survivor." Survivors can be spotted by the large number of service pins they wear. Their motto is always "be safe rather than sorry," and they never make waves or take risks.

The final group are the "effective" followers. Effective followers think and take responsibility for themselves. They are well balanced and possess initiative. If you desire to be a successful nursing professional, you need to become an effective follower and associate only with other effective followers because the influence of the other kinds of followers can negatively affect you and your future.

Develop assertive communication skills so that you feel comfortable communicating needs, desires, and perceptions with your superiors and peers. In many instances, people are stressed and frustrated because they agree to do things that they really do not want to do but feel guilty refusing. You are responsible for communicating your needs and desires. Attend assertiveness training classes, adopt an assertive role model, pray, do whatever you need to do to rid yourself of guilt and the inability to speak up for yourself in an assertive manner. This alone can reduce your daily frustrations and stress.

Be good to yourself. For many nurses, this is a difficult strategy to implement. Traditional female and nursing socialization teaches most nurses to be concerned about other people's comfort and desires. In many instances, this focus leads to deep-seated resentments because no one cares about and for the nurse. These deep-seated resentments can be eliminated by taking total responsibility for being good to yourself rather than waiting for others to be good to you. You can implement this strategy by identifying a specific thing you have always wanted to do or have been jealous of others for being able to do. It could be getting a housekeeper to clean your house, getting your hair or nails done every two weeks, joining a health club, or whatever you would really enjoy doing but have always been reluctant to do because you felt guilty. It is important to get rid of the guilt and to realize that you deserve whatever it is you want. Implementing this strategy can help to alter sacrificing behavior and allow you to take better care of yourself. By being good to yourself, you will improve your attitude and will feel better, work harder, and do what needs to be done to be able to afford bigger and better rewards for yourself. It reverses the tendency to sacrifice oneself for others. You cannot give something to someone else that you do not have yourself. Therefore, you need to be good to yourself before you are even capable of being good to anyone else.

Eliminate whining and complaining from your communication pattern. Whining makes people feel powerless and never really accomplishes anything. Professionals always take responsibility for where they are in their life. If you feel good about yourself but feel that your environment is not providing you with the stimulation, support, satisfaction, and challenge you require, change your environment. You may not be able to change your environment to the extent you need in order to be happy; therefore, the only solution may be to change your attitude and decide to be happy. Whining and complaining only communicate to everyone that you are not in control of your life.

CHALLENGES FOR THE FUTURE

The future is bright and optimistic for the experienced clinical nurse. Professional nurses constitute the largest group of professionals providing health care services. They are the most flexible, have the broadest scope of practice, and have a clinical focus on adaptation to compromised health status that will be the single most important clinical skill in working with an aging population.

The future will also be very challenging for clinical nurses. The delivery of patient care services in hospitals of the future will look very different than it does today as a result of the multiple pressures being placed on all health care providers by the government, consumers, developing technology, and new health care conditions and diseases. Experienced clinical nurses, in conjunction with administrators, must assume their rightful responsibility for developing new organizations and methods to deliver patient care services. As the only on-site clinical experts, experienced nurses are the only people who can truly provide insights into how these challenges can be met while enhancing patient care outcomes.

The entire system of health care delivery will also look very different in the future as a result of numerous hospital professions with overlapping areas of skills who will be competing to obtain their share of limited resources. Experienced clinical nurses must be actively involved in the development of new systems for delivering health care services in our communities. This means that nurses need to be active, volunteering to participate in planning meetings, committee meetings, and so forth, and not to wait until after the fact to complain about decisions made.

In addition to these far-reaching and sometimes overwhelming issues, experienced nurses need to take the leadership role for less experienced and future clinical nurses. They also need drastically to change the way they actualize their professional role by shifting from a mind-set of following policies and procedures and focusing on processes to a focus on planning and evaluating patient care and outcomes. This change in focus has significant implications for the way nurses will operationalize their role as a professional nurse on a daily basis and will have significant and lasting outcomes for patient care.

In some delivery settings, nurses will need to shift their focus from the direct execution of specific tasks and procedures to the supervision of other allied health care professionals performing the tasks. This shift in focus is a result of a decreasing workforce, the escalating salaries of professional nurses, and the declining reimbursement for health care services. To operationalize this role successfully, nurses may need to acquire additional education and experience in supervisory and leadership skills.

Professional nurses will need to focus on managing patient care outcomes by coordinating the efforts and talents of physicians, allied health care workers, and support personnel to set and monitor specific outcomes with specific timeframes for their accomplishment. This will require an ability to plan and evaluate patient responses to specific interventions and make revisions when necessary. It will also force nurses to make more independent decisions on behalf of their patients. In the past, nurses have often waited for others to initiate these decisions and interventions. In the future, they will need to take a more active role in initiating action on behalf of patients. This will stimulate nurses to be more creative in implementing interventions and to acknowledge that there is more than one way to accomplish a specific outcome. The focus on outcomes will stimulate nurses to try alternative interventions or processes when the traditional ones do not produce the desired outcomes.

SUMMARY

As an experienced clinical nurse, it is your responsibility to achieve your own professional satisfaction. This chapter presented a concrete plan of action for experienced nurses to enhance their professional satisfaction. The plan was designed to help you make the decision to take total responsibility for your professional satisfaction, to identify a desired professional goal, and then to actualize that goal through a number of techniques.

The power of the plan and the concepts presented is limited only by the extent to which you implement them and follow through. If you are committed and implement the plan and techniques as presented, the quality of your professional and personal life can be dramatically enhanced.

In continuing or advanced education, the knowledge alone does not provide any rewards or recognition. Professional satisfaction and fulfillment will come only after you take action to implement your newly acquired knowledge.

5

Developing a
Management Self-Image

This chapter assists nurse managers in developing a strong professional self-image to enhance their performance and achievements. It outlines the traditional preparation, education, and socialization of nurse managers and offers strategies for being successful in the role.

The future of the profession is in the hands of nurse leaders. Nurse leaders are nurses in management, executive, research, and clinical roles who are defining and actualizing their desired visions for patient care delivery in their organizations. This chapter specifically focuses on developing the professional self-image of nurse leaders in entry and middle management roles. Chapter six will focus on developing the self-image, performance, and achievements of the nurse executive.

Nurse managers need to focus most of their efforts on becoming exceptional leaders rather than attempting to maintain their clinical expert role. The nurse manager does not practice clinical nursing on a daily basis, so he or she cannot expect or be expected to maintain clinical skills in addition to becoming an exceptional leader. To be a successful nurse manager requires shifting one's focus to developing a vision for nursing, leading and inspiring the staff, and managing oneself. If a nurse manager focuses on maintaining clinical expertise, he or she will fail to assume total responsibility for becoming an expert in leadership and management issues. This usually results in failure in both the clinical and leadership arenas.

KEY CHAPTER CONCEPTS

Key Concept #1

Your self-image is your greatest asset or your greatest liability. A strong self-image is synonymous with self-fulfillment; a weak self-image is synonymous with frustration and burn-out.

Key Concept #2

As a nurse manager, your major role is to be a leader who happens to be a nurse rather than a nurse who happens to be the leader.

Key Concept #3

You must develop a sense of self-confidence, self-discipline, perseverance, tough-mindedness, and the ability to function in a very ambiguous environment to be a successful nurse manager.

Key Concept #4

The most effective strategy for being a successful nurse manager is to be a good role model for all your stakeholders, including your physicians, patients, patients' families, employees, supervisor, and peers. People do not always remember what you say, but they always remember what you do.

Key Concept #5

To be an effective nurse manager, you need to develop skills in financial management, marketing, strategic thinking, political savvy, and personal management.

If you aspire to be or currently are a nurse manager, you must be willing to give up your image as a clinical expert to become a successful nurse leader. The role and responsibility of the nurse manager are very important to the organization and demand your full attention and commitment. Your staff also requires your full leadership time, attention, and commitment.

HISTORICAL SOCIALIZATION OF NURSE MANAGERS

Traditionally, the expert clinical nurse on a unit was chosen to be the leader, or the head nurse, of their unit. They received little management, leadership, or business training or education before assuming the role. In most cases, head nurses were the most technically competent and proficient nurses on the unit. Physicians usually had great respect for them because of their ability to assist the physician.

Most head nurses were trained in the three-year diploma program and were highly socialized in self-discipline and performing according to hospital policies and procedures. They typically focused most of their time and talents working in their clinical area because they were recognized as experts in that area. Head nurses tended to avoid management or administrative functions or tasks because they lacked significant training, experience, and competence in these areas. This encouraged them to maintain the status quo by avoiding change, innovation, and new roles and responsibilities, and it resulted in a lack of competent nursing leaders.

Kramer (1987) reported that nurses recruited by the Magnet hospitals perceived that the effectiveness of their immediate supervisor was very important in the successful retention of nurses. This is good news for the profession because it offers an incentive for more nurse managers to replace their clinical skills with the leadership skills important in making their department, staff nurses, and organization more effective. It can also have a significant and positive impact on organized nursing, patient care delivery, and provider organizations.

It is becoming more common for department directors with strong leadership skills to manage departments that they may not have clinical experience in. These appointments can result in successful outcomes or increased nurse, patient, and physician satisfaction, as well as enhanced financial management of departments based on a cost per unit of service (Strasen, 1987). Other advantages of these appointments are that the leaders focus on their leadership role and responsibilities and acknowledge that the clinical experts are the ones that provide actual patient care. When clinical issues require operational decisions, the leader is forced to involve the staff in making these decisions and policies. As a result, the nursing staff feels that they have a strong involvement in decision-making in their immediate work unit. This kind of leadership calls for a more egalitarian approach to the management and operation of a nursing unit. It communicates that a department is a team of professionals working together in different roles and capacities to provide quality care and service at a predetermined cost rather than a group of subordinates working for a superior who directs their actions.

The traditional head nurse role is changing in response to the scaling down of health care organizations and the need to respond in a more timely manner to stakeholders. In many hospitals, the director of nursing has been upgraded to a member of the executive management team. Because the scope and responsibility of the director of nursing is increasing, the scope and responsibility of the nurse manager role is also changing. These changes involve risk and uncertainty for incumbents and new nurse managers. Some incumbents find these trends threatening; others find them exciting and challenging. Ultimately, the influence of the nurse manager in administrative and operational decision-making will have a positive and enhancing effect on the entire nursing staff of an organization and will upgrade the image of the entire profession, as well as improving the delivery of patient care.

As the nurse manager role changes, the skills and education required for this role will also change. It is very important for existing and aspiring nurse managers to understand these changes completely. If you are an aspiring nurse manager, you must understand what the role requires. Your expectations for the role must be clear and accurate or you will experience role conflict and ambiguity, which have been cited as major causes of stress and burn-out for nurse leaders.

If you are currently a nurse manager, you probably have experienced frustration and stress because the role you are in today is very different from what it was a few months or years ago. It is important to develop a clear understanding of the magnitude and direction of the changes in the role so that you can make appropriate decisions for your future career.

Nurse managers need to devote long hours of hard work to be

successful. Therefore, it is essential that they enjoy what they are doing. If they do not, they will not perform to or achieve their maximum potential. It is very important to identify what you enjoy doing and to plan your career accordingly. If you are a nurse manager but do not enjoy your work, find a role that you can enjoy and develop a plan to attain that role. Otherwise, you are likely to do a mediocre job, and your staff may pick up this standard and also do a mediocre job, and the quality and level of patient care on your unit will be compromised. If you are in such a situation, it is your responsibility to change your role for the benefit of all your stakeholders.

For the benefit of the profession, nurses that do not enjoy their work need to find a role or position they can enjoy. If they cannot find such a role in nursing, they do the entire profession and their patients a disservice by continuing to go through the motions and spreading their unhappiness, disenchantment, and frustration. Their negativity will have a significant negative effect on new nurses, potential nurses, patients and their families, and the entire image of the profession. This is true even with a nursing shortage; a smaller number of positive, enthusiastic nurses can provide higher quality of care than an adequate number of burned-out, negative, frustrated nurses.

SELF-IMAGE AND
THE NURSE MANAGER ROLE

Your self-image drastically affects your performance and achievements and is very important to being a successful nurse manager. As a nurse manager, your self-image is your greatest asset or your greatest liability *(Key Concept #4)*. A strong self-image is synonymous with self-fulfillment; a weak self-image is synonymous with frustration and burn-out. Research has shown that managers with high self-esteem work harder in response to difficult goals than managers with low self-esteem (Carroll & Tosi, 1970). People with high self-esteem are more apt to respond to failure situations with increased persistence because of their strong confidence in their abilities. Their abilities and self-confidence in turn result in successful outcomes (Brockner & Rubin, 1985).

When faced with problems, people who are not confident in their own abilities quit sooner because they do not believe that they have the talent and ability to overcome them. They may have the ability to solve the problems; however, because they do not believe they have the ability, they do not exhibit it.

Middle managers with a high level of self-esteem adapt better to a rapidly changing environment and the resulting role requirements than those with low self-esteem (Morrison, 1977). Managers with high self-esteem exhibit a more open belief system that allows them to adapt better to change. Managers with low self-esteem have difficulty adapting or functioning in a changing environment because they question their ability to function in a stable, rigid environment. When their environment changes, they become very threatened and stressed because of their limited belief in their own abilities.

The most effective strategy for being a successful nurse manager is to be a good role model for all your stakeholders *(Key Concept #2)*. This concept is important because employees with low self-esteem are more highly influenced by the behavior of their role models than high self-esteem employees (Bandura, 1977). Because of their insecurities, people with low self-esteem act like their leaders or role models. As a leader, it is therefore very important to be a good role model because of the influence you have on people in your work group. Role modeling is an important leadership strategy and skill to positively influence people in a specific work group.

A field study by Mossholder, Bedian, and Armenakis (1981) explored the effects of self-esteem and peer group interaction on the propensity to leave a job, work performance, and job tension. Their results showed that nurses with low self-esteem performed better when their interaction with their peer group was high. However, the performance of nurses with high self-esteem was not affected by their level of peer group interaction. These results indicate that the performance of a nursing department is affected by the level of self-esteem of the nurses as well as by their peer group interaction. This provides valuable information to help nurse managers create a work environment that will enhance employee performance. If your nurses have a low level of self-esteem, group interaction is a key motivating force for them. However, if you have a group of nurses who have a high level of self-esteem, they do not necessarily need peer interaction or pressure to perform on a specific level.

As a nurse leader, you need to structure the interactions among peers on your unit to create a positive influence on them. If peer group interaction on a unit supports negativity, burn-out, and performing in a mediocre way, it becomes a powerful influence on the behavior and performance of your nurses with low-esteem. If you have a large number of nurses with low self-esteem, you can enhance their performance by being a positive role model and encouraging peer interactions that promote quality patient care outcomes, a positive, "can-do" attitude, and a commitment to excellence.

Research has also shown that nurses with low self-esteem exhibit significantly lower job satisfaction and performance in the presence of role ambiguity and role conflict than do nurses with high self-esteem (Mossholder, Bedian, & Armenakis, 1981). Nurses with low self-esteem are more comfortable in very stable and routine environments in which they need to make few decisions. Nurses with high self-esteem, however, perform better in participatory management environments in which they are actively involved in departmental decision-making.

These research findings on self-esteem can explain why some nursing units respond very well to the changes presently occurring in health care while others do not. They also explain why some nursing units respond very well to a decentralized, participative model of operating, while others prefer to function in a more traditional, bureaucratic operational style. As a nurse manager, it is your responsibility to enhance the self-image and self-esteem of your staff to function in a decentralized, unit-based management system in which all professionals contribute to the decisions made on behalf of the unit and the patients. In an environment of declining resources, all professionals on a unit need to contribute actively to decisions about how resources are allocated to ensure quality outcomes. However, before this can happen on a broad scale, the self-image and self-esteem of individual nurses must be enhanced.

Low employee self-esteem has numerous other implications for the effective functioning of a unit that must be responded to by the nurse manager. Brockner (1988) identified the following four examples of employee behavior resulting from low self-esteem that is detrimental to the organization.

First, some employees are reluctant to seek assistance from others when they have problems performing. Asking for help from others requires a fairly positive and strong self-image. When employees have problems performing but do not ask for help, patient outcomes may be compromised.

Second, employees with low self-esteem are unwilling to negotiate or compromise with peers in difficult situations because they feel that it will appear that they have given in or failed. This unwillingness to negotiate may create problems of cooperation in the organization.

Third, employees or managers with low self-esteem are reluctant to withdraw from a project that is really a losing proposition because of their own personal insecurities. Their commitment to the losing proposition may lead to losses that could be preventable. Employees with high self-esteem can usually let go of projects that are evaluated as a failure without becoming personally threatened.

Fourth, employees with low self-esteem usually perform at suboptimal levels because peers and superiors have low expectations for their performance. People perform at the level of expectation set for them by themselves or others.

The more a person's work role requires the person to act in a manner consistent with high self-esteem, the greater their self-esteem actually becomes (Kohn & Schooler, 1983). This means that as a manager you can make an impact on the self-esteem of your employees by expecting them to act in ways consistent with having a high level of self-esteem.

The influence of role modeling is key in the performance of any work group. Employees role model the self-esteem level of their leaders just as children role model the self-esteem of their mothers (Brockner, 1988). One study referred to this concept as "basking in reflected glory" and suggested that the role modeling of self-esteem influences people to the degree that they feel connected to their role model (Cialdini & Richardson, 1980). Likewise, if the leader has a low level of self-esteem, subordinates may role model poor behaviors and performance to the degree they feel connected to the leader.

The self-esteem of an employee is also directly related to his or her performance appraisals. As a manager and leader you are a very credible source of feedback for your employees. You may not always be in touch with the high credibility you have with your staff; however, even though employees may consciously discount your feedback, they are usually very affected by it. Therefore, it is important that you provide employees with responsible feedback in an acceptable and timely manner.

Negative feedback given in person or through performance appraisals usually has a more adverse effect on the future performance of people with low self-esteem than on those with high self-esteem (Brockner, Derr & Laing, 1987). People with low self-esteem usually respond to constructive feedback with defensive and blaming behavior because they need to defend or protect their low self-esteem from further blows or attempts to discredit them. This kind of defensive behavior is very common among nurses. As a nurse leader, you need to

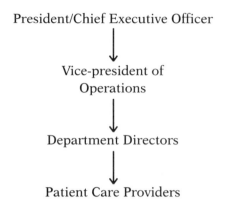

President/Chief Executive Officer

Vice-president of
Operations

Department Directors

Patient Care Providers

Figure 5-1. Organizational Structure for the 1990s Hospital

bolster your staff's self-confidence by verbalizing your confidence in their abilities and setting goals and expectations of excellence for their actions rather than defending their actions.

THE CHANGING ORGANIZATION

Tom Peters, in his salient book *Thriving on Chaos* (1987), states that organizational structures and management tactics need to change drastically to respond to an environment of fast-paced innovation. He directs organizations to reduce their bureaucratic hierarchies to a total of three to five management layers, with minimum spans of control of twenty-five to seventy-five employees per manager. He believes that workplace communication patterns need to shift from vertical communication to horizontal communication or communication between functional departments. This horizontal communication needs to focus on constantly improving the service being provided.

According to Peters, the ideal organizational structure for a successful hospital in this changing environment will resemble that shown in Figure 5-1. This downsized organizational structure has four levels and is appropriate for hospitals with 100 to 350 beds. Hospitals with more than 350 beds may need an additional layer of management or more than one vice-president. Small departments that typically have fewer than ten employees will be combined into larger departments that will be cross-trained to perform multiple functions with multiple skills. These multiskilled workers will be paid higher salaries. Their increased job variety and higher salaries will result in increased job satisfaction. For example, most hospitals have individual pulmonary, respiratory therapy, cardiology, and neurology departments. These could be combined to form a multiple-service ancillary department under the direction of a generalist leader or department manager. Shift supervisors will be cross-trained to perform multiple functions and will be working supervisors who will maintain their clinical skills. Department managers will have twenty-four-hour accountability for departmental operations and will not be able to maintain their expert clinical skills because of their larger span of control and administrative focus.

NEW ROLE AND RESPONSIBILITIES

The new nurse manager or department director role is the most important role in the successful health care organization of the future. It is similar to the role of chief operating officer for a specific product or service line. The nursing department director orchestrates the efforts of a number of disciplines to ensure that a high level of quality and service is being provided to patients at a cost that will maintain organizational viability or profitability.

The role of department manager requires direct communication with all stakeholders. The department manager meets frequently with stakeholders to brainstorm and implement ways to improve patient care delivery. Display 5-1 contrasts the new nurse manager role with the traditional head nurse role.

According to **Key Concept #5,** you need basic education in business and leadership skills to be a successful nurse manager in this changing environment (Strasen, 1987). Abilities that will assist you to be a successful nurse manager in the future include:

1. An ability to role model the values of your organization 365 days a year.
2. An ability to envision your desired future for your unit and communicate that vision to your stakeholders.
3. An ability to lead your staff to your desired vision for your unit.

Display 5-1
THE SHIFTING FOCUS OF THE
NURSE MANAGER ROLE

Focus of *Head Nurse Role*	*Focus of Department* *Manager Role*
Support and defend nursing care	Challenge staff to exceed past performances
Focus on correct process	Focus on excellent outcomes
Closely supervise nurses	Lead employees to vision
Protect departmental boundaries	Eliminate departmental boundaries
Receive direction and approval from above	Negotiate operational changes needed with peers
Standardization across nursing units	Each operating unit designs operations around its unique stakeholders
Focus on the clinical supervision of nurses	Focus on total management of the service provided to maximize stakeholder satisfaction at the lowest cost
Expert in clinical practice	Leader in the operation of a business unit
Communicate by memo	Frequently communicate in person
Ensure that policies and procedures are followed	Act in the best interests of all stakeholders and change policies and procedures to reflect those interests

(continued)

Display 5-1 *(continued)*
THE SHIFTING FOCUS OF THE
NURSE MANAGER ROLE

Focus of *Head Nurse Role*	*Focus of Department* *Manager Role*
Policeman	Facilitator
Mother	Mentor
Maintain stability	Promote change
Reward employees for longevity	Reward employees for performance, outcomes, and innovation
Rewarded for stability, process, and longevity	Rewarded for innovation, outcomes, and execution

---

4. An ability to manage yourself physically and emotionally.
5. An ability to quantify your ideas about quality and cost of nursing care.
6. An ability to role model a love of change.
7. An ability to respond proactively to an ambiguous health care environment.
8. An ability to foster innovation in your staff.
9. Excellent time-management skills.
10. An ability to maintain a good sense of humor.
11. An ability to think and act strategically.

As a nurse manager, you will assume responsibility for larger numbers of employees. If your hospital has small nursing units, you will be responsible for multiple units. The number of beds you will be responsible for will vary based on staffing ratios, which are determined by the level of service being provided. For example, as a critical care department manager, you will be responsible for fewer beds than a department director of a medical surgical unit. Typically, a nurse manager's responsibility will include forty to seventy-five employees and fifty to sixty medical surgical beds, twenty to forty intensive care beds, or thirty to fifty intermediate care beds.

As a nurse manager, your role will expand to manage professionals and ancillary staff from many different disciplines. Your staff may include dietary employees, housekeeping employees, secretaries, respiratory therapists, physical therapy staff, financial counselors, case managers, utilization review nurses, and infection control nurses. You will need to expand your leadership and managerial focus to include a wide range of employees of different skill levels who have multi-disciplinary perspectives.

In this type of health care environment, you will need to be comfortable giving up your hard-earned clinical skills for skills in leadership and business and make the transition from a nurse who happens to be a manager or leader to a manager or leader who happens to be a nurse *(Key Concept #2)*. This is a very difficult transition for many nurses to make, and some never actually make the transition. Others believe it is not a necessary or desirable transition to make. However, it is not only a desirable transition but also a crucial one that must be made if you are to be successful in your leadership role.

As a nursing department manager, you will lead and supervise all employees who provide a direct service to patients or a support service to a specific unit. You will be expected to collaborate with the direct care or service providers in order to enhance the service and care delivered by incorporating the customer's perspectives, needs, and wants into the delivery of the service. Display 5-2 lists a number of key attitudes and abilities you must develop to be successful in this role.

As a nurse manager, your stakeholders are defined in a much larger context than the traditional head nurse role. To be effective and successful, you will need constantly to listen to and balance the numerous and sometimes conflicting needs and wants of your stakeholders. Your stakeholders include your patients and their families, your physicians, your employees, regulatory and accreditation agencies, the media, your peers, your superiors, and professional colleagues outside of your organization.

As a clinical nurse, your stakeholders were limited to patients, physicians, patients' families, and your head nurse. In almost all cases, the needs and wants of these stakeholders are very similar and can be generalized as quality care provided in a timely and courteous manner.

Display 5-2
KEY ATTITUDES AND ABILITIES FOR
THE SUCCESSFUL NURSE MANAGER

1. An ability to lead by role modeling and interacting with all stakeholders on an ongoing basis to improve the care and service provided.
2. An ability to role model the love of change on a daily basis in order to respond to the ever-changing needs and wants of stakeholders.
3. An ability to implement many pilot projects simultaneously to improve daily unit operations.
4. An ability to challenge and channel all employees to identify, support, and implement innovative ways of performing their jobs to improve the department.
5. An ability constantly to recognize and give credit to employees for their contributions and ideas, no matter how small or large they are.
6. An ability to listen to all stakeholders for ways to improve the product and operations without getting defensive.
7. An ability to maintain a positive, "can do" attitude at all times.
8. An ability and desire to coach and develop the staff to be the best they can be.

As you move away from the bedside, your stakeholders increase in number and in the diversity of their needs and wants. Because of this diversity of interests, decision-making becomes more political and less clinical. Figure 5-2 depicts the shift from clinical to political decision-making as the number of stakeholders increases.

The downsizing and reduction in the hierarchy of organizations in the late 1980s resulted in an average of two levels of management above the nurse manager. This reduction in the number of superiors places the nurse manager much closer to the political arena. This is where political battles are fought because a decision to satisfy one

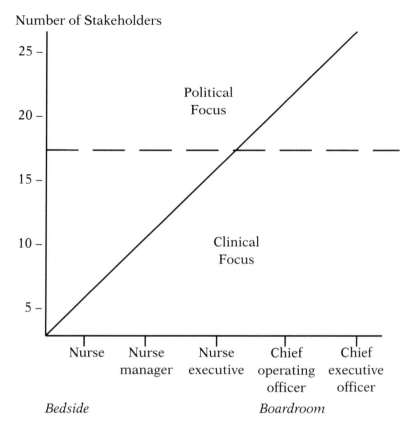

Figure 5-2. Nature of Decision-Making in Hospitals

group of stakeholders negatively affects other groups of stakeholders. In the new nurse manager role, you need to develop an ability to balance the multiple and conflicting needs and wants of your stakeholders without jeopardizing your position in the process. When decentralization and downsizing encourage operational decisions to be made on the departmental level rather than by the nurse executive or the chief executive officer, you will need to develop the political savvy and skills to make those decisions.

For example, imagine that you are the nurse manager on a cardiac floor. Your top admitting cardiologist makes rounds at 6:00 A.M. daily (three out of five days it is actually 7:00 A.M., but you never know when those days are!) and demands that the daily weights be documented on the patient care record by that time. The 11:00 P.M. to 7:00 A.M. nursing staff has had difficulty getting the weights recorded between the hours of five and six. Your patients have been complaining to you and documenting in the patient satisfaction survey that the care they receive on your unit is wonderful, but that they cannot understand why they are awakened at 5:30 A.M. to be weighed. How do you resolve this issue and keep your patients, nurses, and physicians happy?

This is an example of an operational decision that needs to be made on a unit level. It is crucial to resolve the issue and accomplish your goal of maximizing the satisfaction of all three of your stakeholders. A number of potential solutions for this problem would meet with positive support from some of your stakeholders but may be strongly opposed by others. The trick is to come up with a solution that will meet some of the needs of all your stakeholders without alienating any specific individual or group. This is not always easy, and it is really a political decision rather than a clinical decision.

Decisions that are made in the political arena on the graph in Figure 5-2 constitute a gray zone. This means that there really is no right or wrong solution to the problem. However, your stakeholders believe that the decisions are black and white because they want you to make the decision they recommend. When large numbers of stakeholders are involved, management decisions become highly political because you are dealing with multiple consequences for each perspective that each stakeholder holds.

Historically, these decisions and policies were made by the nurse executive for the entire nursing department. Head nurses would respond to all their stakeholders by simply saying, for instance, "I'm sorry but our policy is that we weigh all patients between 6:30 A.M. and 7:30 A.M." The head nurse was off the hook and although the stakeholders may have been upset, they learned to live with the policy because they didn't see any alternative.

In the new role of the nurse manager, you do not have the luxury of falling back on an unreasonable system with unreasonable rules. You will need to make these difficult decisions yourself and then learn to live with them. You will actually make better decisions, but you will personally be more at risk in your management role. You are likely to get the blame when anything goes wrong, but you will rarely get the credit for good decisions. As a nurse manager, you will need to be prepared emotionally and have the skills to assume this kind of responsibility and accountability.

Jan Carlzon, the chief executive of SAS Airlines, described the manager as the person who actively seeks out ways to make daily operations occur more efficiently. Managers are expected to tear down the traditional barriers that occur between departments on behalf of the product or service being provided (Carlzon, 1987). Peters calls this "horizontal barrier bashing" and believes that this is where organizations will gain the most efficiency in their operations in the next decade.

A number of inefficiencies occur at the boundaries between traditional hospital functions and departments. For example, two or more departments may duplicate efforts (i.e., respiratory therapy personnel and nursing staff both documenting respirator settings). Increased and repetitive communication may be needed between staff in nursing and the ancillary departments because of the highly specialized and fragmented nature of the ancillary departments.

Fragmented distribution of supplies and labor to patients may result from large centralized ancillary and support departments such as central supply or pharmacy.

As a nurse manager, you will be the on-call expert to assist your staff in delivering patient care services. You must be sure you have trained, equipped, and socialized your staff to be able to provide the quality and level of service that is expected by your patients, patients' families, and physicians. As the nurse manager, you must ensure that your staff is able to evaluate the service they provide, and able to identify and implement new and better ways for providing services to your physicians, patients, and patients' families. You must continuously look for ways to improve your own departmental operations and outcomes. In this role, you will function as a trainer, evaluator, systems analyst, cheerleader, marketer, etc.

THE NEW LEADERSHIP STYLE

The management traits and skills for success in the future require you to adopt a very different set of assumptions about yourself, your staff, and your organization. Display 5-3 contrasts traditional and new leadership assumptions.

To be an effective and successful nurse manager, you will need to develop a willingness and ability to lead by example, to delegate, and to defer decision-making on departmental issues to your staff. This

Display 5-3
TRADITIONAL AND
NEW LEADERSHIP ASSUMPTIONS

Traditional Nursing Management Assumptions	New Leadership Assumptions
Nursing must be closely supervised to maintain good clinical outcomes.	Peer review can enhance clinical outcomes.
My role is to make decisions.	My role is to facilitate decision-making by listening to all the stakeholders.
I determine the staffing patterns and model of care.	I facilitate the development and implementation of the model of care and staffing patterns based on feedback from physicians, nurses, patients, and patients' families.
I make decisions based on what my boss thinks I should do.	I make decisions based on feedback from all my stakeholders.
I communicate mostly vertically with my subordinates and boss.	I spend most of my time communicating horizontally with my peers to overcome traditional functional barriers to providing good patient care.
I am compensated for being a nurse who happens to know some management theories and applications.	I am compensated for being a leader of a business unit that is striving to maximize stakeholder satisfaction at the most efficient cost.

requires an ability to give up some of the traditional management tasks and practices and to assume additional risk by involving your staff in decision-making. It is easier to make all the decisions yourself and communicate them by memo to your staff than it is to allow your stakeholders to make recommendations on issues that they are closely involved in and then change or implement the systems to make those recommendations a reality. In most instances, the best ideas for improving patient care or reducing costs mandate that you negotiate with other department directors or with senior management, or try to change existing policies, procedures, or traditional ways of doing things in your organization. Involving direct care staff always results in better decisions but will usually include additional risk for you as the leader. This is the role and responsibility of the new nurse manager. You need to ask yourself, Is this for me?

RISKS OF NURSE MANAGEMENT

The nurse manager role is significantly increasing in formal power and authority as well as overall accountability. There are some increased risks for the role that need to be understood clearly before you set a goal to be a nurse manager. Corporate takeovers, mergers of independent health care organizations, and the drastic changes occurring in the health care industry produce greater risk for all nursing roles other than that of direct care providers.

In this environment, you must develop a strong and positive self-image and sense of self-worth to survive the downsizing, resizing, reorganization, and turmoil that frequently results in voluntary and involuntary terminations. As a nurse in a management or executive role, you must be emotionally and financially ready and able to change jobs and roles or be terminated on very short notice without feeling that you are a failure. It is a traumatic experience to have your job eliminated through downsizing or to be asked to leave because of philosophical differences when you have a strong and positive professional self-image. The experience can be devastating if you lack a strong professional self-image. You must be able to separate what happens politically in the organization from who you are personally and professionally and realize that termination may have nothing to do with who you are or what you have done or not done.

The farther away from the bedside you get, the less job security you have. If you want to proceed on a nursing leadership career path, you must prepare yourself to be fired at any time. This preparation has an economic and an emotional component. Preparing yourself economically includes the ability to survive financially for one to three months without a salary.

If your job is eliminated, you may actually receive anywhere from one to three months' severance pay, depending on individual circumstances. However, in cases in which you choose to resign you may not get anything. If you are not economically prepared to leave at any time, you may be put in a position in which you are forced to do something you do not feel comfortable with to meet your financial obligations.

The second aspect of preparing for termination is being emotionally able to separate your professional and personal self from the act of being terminated. Many nurses feel that the worst thing that could happen to them in their professional careers is to be fired. As a nurse manager, you will need to understand that you operate in a very political environment.

To be a successful nurse manager, you need to develop political savvy. This means learning to say the right thing to the right person most of the time. If you are good leader, however, there is a high probability that sometime you will say the wrong thing to the wrong person at the wrong time. When that happens, you may be fired. This does not mean that you are incompetent, unintelligent, unprofessional, or a bad person. It only means that you are a leader who said the wrong thing to the wrong person at the wrong time.

If you can emotionally internalize this thinking and save at least three months' salary or benefits you can and will survive being fired. Not only will you survive the experience, you will learn many valuable lessons that will help you perform better in the future. You will also be a much stronger leader and person for having gone through the experience. Remember the old adage, "no pain, no gain."

On the other hand, if you do not take steps to prepare yourself emotionally and economically to be terminated at any time, the experience potentially can destroy your future career. If you do not prepare yourself emotionally and if you do get fired, your mind will start telling you that you are a bad person, incompetent, unprofessional, ineffective, and a poor manager and nurse. According to the psychocybernetic model, you will act in accordance with all these thoughts and beliefs.

When you interview for your next job, you will behave in ways that are consistent with your thoughts and you will come across as incompetent, unprofessional, and ineffective. If you act this way in an interview, you will not get the job and your future career will be hampered. Therefore, you need to prepare yourself for potential termination before the fact, so that if you get fired you can immediately go into your preprogrammed attitude that you are a great leader who just happened to be in the wrong place at the wrong time and said the wrong thing to the wrong person. If you have developed this attitude, your career will not be negatively affected by the incident.

There are a number of specific actions you can take to prepare yourself for potential termination. Acknowledge that the environment of management is politically charged. There is a high level of probability that you or your job could be eliminated or reassigned. As a successful nurse leader, you may say the wrong thing to the wrong person at the wrong time and be asked to leave.

Understand and internalize that when you find yourself in this position, it does not mean that you are an incompetent nurse, incompetent leader, or a bad person. It just means that you had a goal and tried to sell the wrong goal to the wrong person at the wrong time.

Discuss the risk of being fired or laid off with your significant other. Acknowledge that you both must be emotionally and economically prepared for this possibility. By having this discussion in a planning situation rather than in a crisis situation, you will not alienate one another at a time when you need each other's support.

Develop and practice your speech for two to three months' severance pay that you will give immediately when you are asked to leave. All organizations will give you at least two weeks' pay. They also would prefer that you leave quietly, and many would be willing to pay two to three months' salary just to have you leave quietly without retaining a lawyer. If you do not ask for things, you will not get them. Therefore, be prepared to deliver the speech the moment you receive notification of your termination. If you deliver the speech a day or week later, you have no bargaining clout at all. This speech is only to be delivered if you have not been grossly neglectful in your duties. If that is the case, you should just leave quietly.

Develop and implement a plan to save enough vacation time or money for your family to exist comfortably without your salary for two to three months. This action will decrease the stress on you and your family while you look for another position if you are terminated. It will give you the freedom to look for the role you want rather than just taking the first job that comes along.

Establish a personal relationship with a professional search firm while you are still employed and happy with your current job. You never know when things can change, and search firms do not go out of their way to market people who are out of work the first time they meet them. You need to establish this relationship when you are successfully functioning in a responsible role rather than when you are in between opportunities.

EXPECTATIONS DETERMINE PERFORMANCE

The Pygmalion effect is used to describe the situation in which the expectations of a leader determine how subordinates perform. According to Greek mythology, King Pygmalion of Cyprus sculpted his version of the perfect woman in ivory and then fell in love with the sculpture. Aphrodite, the goddess of love, then gave life to Pygmalion's statue. The moral behind the myth is that you get what you expect to get. If you expect that your employees will perform poorly or that they will fail, you communicate that message to them through your behavior, and they will perform poorly. On the other hand, if you expect them to be productive, innovative, and successful and rise to challenging situations, their performance will match your expectations.

Rosenthal and Jacobson (1968) have done many studies in this area with college students. They identified the self-fulfilling prophecy, or theory that the achievements of students have less to do with their ability than with the teacher's expectations of how students will perform. This theory has significant application in the business world. When a leader or manager believes and expects employees to perform on a high level, they do perform on a high level and perceive their jobs as more satisfying and rewarding because of their high performance.

As a nurse manager, it is crucial that you consistently expect your staff to do their best in providing quality care and service to patients, physicians, patients' families, and one another. Sometimes (or many times), individual nurses will disappoint you and perform lower than your expectations or their abilities. In these cases, intervene directly and in a timely manner, but never let the individual cases interfere with your overall optimistic and high expectations for your staff. If you allow individual nurses or situations to lower your overall expectations for your staff as a group, your staff will lower their standards to match your expectations.

DEVELOPING A MANAGEMENT SELF-IMAGE

When people think about the image of a manager, they have some common assumptions about how people in management positions look, talk, walk, and think. Those common management expectations or assumptions include:

- Managers are intelligent.
- Managers are self-controlled.
- Managers have good people skills.
- Managers appear neat and well-groomed.
- Managers juggle numerous different tasks and situations at once.
- Managers are responsible people.
- Managers work long hours.
- Managers can get the answers to all your questions.
- Managers have the ability to get things done.

Any strategy to develop or enhance your self-image as a nurse manager begins by focusing on incorporating these traits and characteristics in your own self-image. Your plan to become a successful nurse manager needs to include setting a professional goal to become a nurse manager, developing short-term objectives to get to that goal, developing and repeating positive affirmations to program your self-image to attain the goal and objectives, and visualizing yourself as a nurse manager.

Step One:
Take Responsibility for the
Nurse Manager Goal

The first step in becoming a nurse manager is to develop a strong desire to become one and to make a conscious choice to pay the price of attaining that goal. The nurse manager role is very challenging and you cannot make a commitment to it without fully understanding the benefits and difficulties of the role.

There are many nurse managers who entered the role more than five years ago and who are currently very unhappy and frustrated. The role they entered five years ago was very different from the role they are experiencing today. If you are one of these managers, you need to clarify your role and responsibilities. If you do not enjoy them, then you should get out of the role as soon as possible. You are not a failure if this is how you feel. You are simply acknowledging that the role has changed significantly, that you do not enjoy the new role, and that you owe it to yourself to be happy in your professional career.

Step Two:
Define Your Professional Management Goal

Write your specific professional goal down on paper, in the present tense, and with a specific deadline.

If the nurse manager role sounds challenging and stimulating and you have made a decision to commit yourself to attaining the role, you need to develop a two-year goal for the specific management role you desire. Do you want to be a nurse manager in your existing hospital? In a community hospital? In a university hospital? In a large hospital or a small facility? In a for-profit or not-for-profit organization? Do you want to be a nurse manager in your clinical specialty or in a completely different area of specialization? Are you seeking your first management job or, if you have functioned successfully in a management role, are you seeking a middle-manager role?

Define your desired management role as specifically and precisely as possible, including the type of health care organization, the level of the management role, and the general location of the organization. A sample professional management goal would be: *By* _____ , *19___ , I am the nurse manager of the emergency department in my current hospital.*

Step Three:
Management Self-Assessment

The next step in accomplishing your nurse manager goal is to complete a management self-assessment. It is important to complete this self-assessment to identify the major areas on which you need to focus to attain your desired professional goal in the next two years. Display 5-4 outlines specific management criteria with the ideal management self-image for each of the criteria. In the middle column, write an assessment of your existing self-image in relation to the criteria outlined in the left-hand column. By comparing your current self-assessment in the middle column with the ideal management self-image outlined in the right-hand column, you can identify the areas on which you need to focus your short-term objectives.

Step Four:
Develop Short-Term Objectives

After completing your nurse manager self-assessment, develop three short-term objectives that you can accomplish in one year based on the discrepancies between your current self-image and your desired management self-image. Display 5-5 (p. 137) provides you with some sample short-term objectives that can be accomplished in one year to move you closer to your professional management goal.

Step Five:
Program Yourself for Your
Management Role

The two methods for reprogramming your self-image to accomplish your professional goals are positive affirmations and visualization. After you have identified your desired management role, find or create a picture of yourself in this desired role and put the picture on your refrigerator so that you can reprogram your self-image daily. Make sure the picture depicts exactly the way you desire to be perceived by others and the way you will appear as a nurse manager. There are many different messages you communicate through your personal appearance and dress. Before deciding on a specific physical appearance, consider the implications outlined in Display 5-6 (pp. 138–139).

Develop at least one positive affirmation for each objective based on the guidelines covered in Chapter Three. Display 5-7 (p. 140) provides a sample list of positive affirmations for specific short-term objectives to attain a nurse manager role.

(text continues on page 136)

Display 5-4
NURSE MANAGER SELF-ASSESSMENT

Management Characteristics	Your Current Self-Image	Ideal Management Self-Image
Graduate education		Master's degree
Knowledge of nursing issues, leadership issues, hospital financial issues, reimbursement issues, Joint Commission of Accreditation of Healthcare Organizations (JCAHO) issues, licensing issues, medical staff issues, health care industry issues, and basic business skills		Broad overview of key nursing, hospital, and financial reimbursement issues; in-depth knowledge of licensing and JCAHO issues
Business attire		Business suit, slacks, or dresses with or without a lab coat; closed toe pumps; no low-cut necklines
Classic jewelry		Classic gold or silver pieces; no dangling earrings
Briefcase		Black, brown, or burgundy leather briefcase
Purse		Small and organized; when carrying a purse and briefcase, purse needs to fit inside the briefcase

Display 5-4 *(continued)*
NURSE MANAGER SELF-ASSESSMENT

Management Characteristics	Your Current Self-Image	Ideal Management Self-Image
Political savvy		Beginning understanding of who to say what to and when; knowledge of who has the informal power and how to make the boss look good
Self-control		Never cry or appear tired or overwhelmed in public
Time-management skills		Learn how to get the important things done before deadlines
		Learn to do more than one thing at a time
		Learn to stop doing things that do not make a difference
Need for recognition		Satisfaction with recognition from boss; able to give credit to staff for departmental accomplishments
Ability to sell ideas		Beginning selling skills
Vision		Be able to implement vision of top management

(continued)

Display 5-4 *(continued)*
NURSE MANAGER SELF-ASSESSMENT

Management Characteristics	Your Current Self-Image	Ideal Management Self-Image
Management self-image		See yourself as capable of handling most difficult situations or know where to get help to deal with issues; see yourself as a manager that happens to be a nurse
Assertive communication		Able to give and receive constructive feedback in a direct, nondefensive manner
Response to high-risk environment		Emotionally and economically prepared to be fired at any time
Response to ambiguous environment		Learn to love change

STRATEGIES FOR EXCELLENCE

This section lists a number of strategies for becoming an excellent nurse manager that I have learned from my colleagues, research in the field, world leaders, books, tapes, and personal experiences.

Take one action step today to accomplish one of your short-term objectives. Actions you might take include sending for information brochures on graduate education programs, going shopping to purchase a new outfit, or going to a beauty salon to get your hair done in a style more appropriate for a manager.

Display 5-5
SHORT-TERM MANAGEMENT OBJECTIVES

1. By _____ , 19 _____ ,
   I have enrolled in a graduate program.

2. By _____ , 19 _____ ,
   I have a mentor.

3. By _____ , 19 _____ ,
   I have completed a management class.

4. By _____ , 19 _____ ,
   I have developed a written plan for becoming a nurse manager
   within the next two years.

Approach a nurse manager you respect from your organization or another organization to share your management goal with and to ask for assistance in attaining your goal. Most nurse managers are very flattered when another nurse asks them for professional career counseling or an ongoing mentor relationship. This action communicates to the mentor that he or she has done something memorable to gain your admiration. Nurse managers are usually very happy to give career advice on a one-time or ongoing basis.

Develop a sense of perseverance toward your goal to be a nurse manager. You can develop this by faithfully repeating your positive affirmations and visualizing your nurse manager role.

Learn to act quickly and decisively. If you keep up on current knowledge in the field, your decisions will be on target and you will not have to hesitate to analyze things in order to be accurate.

Develop a habit of looking for others and yourself doing things right, and then acknowledge them. By noting other people doing things right, you will automatically become a hero because you will help them to develop a positive self-image.

Imagine that you are constantly being videotaped and tape

Display 5-6
IMAGE IMPLICATIONS

Physical Appearance	Message Communicated/ Implications
White uniform	The nurse manager that wears white communicates a focus on patient care and being one of the clinical nursing staff. Stakeholders tend to expect the manager to perform the same tasks as direct care givers when the manager wears white.
Dress or slacks with lab coat	Street clothes worn with a lab coat communicate a management role with a clinical focus. The lab coat communicates an authority figure and distances one from the staff, which is an effective management strategy for many situations.

(continued)

recorded while you are within the walls of your organization. If you pretend this, you will consistently role model all the behaviors and words that are appropriate for you as an influential role model for your employees. As a leader, you must believe and behave as though you have the responsibility to role model the expected actions and words all of the time. This is easy if you imagine that you are always being watched. In reality, you are being watched constantly by your employees, and your actions always speak louder than your words.

Be willing and able to give up being right to accomplish specific objectives. As a nurse manager, you are operating in a political rather than clinical environment. In most situations, people will help you to achieve your objectives if they are involved in the process or if they get

Display 5-6 *(continued)*
IMAGE IMPLICATIONS

Physical Appearance	Message Communicated/ Implications
Business attire	The nurse manager in business attire communicates a more administrative role and responsibility that is consistent with the new nurse manager. Business attire encourages physicians to relate to the nurse manager on a peer level and adds credibility to decisions made by the manager in front of physicians, patients, and staff. Physicians tend to be uncomfortable with nurse managers dressed in business attire and may kid them about not really working. Staff nurses may feel rejected or abandoned by the nurse manager in business attire and feel that the manager will not be available to assist them. These feelings usually disappear when the nurse manager role models high visibility and increased authority, and when the manager is available to staff irrespective of clothing worn.

credit for an idea or recognition for providing you with the right answer. If you have a strong desire to be right in your dealings with physicians, administrators, or your boss, many times you will lose, because they need to save face themselves.

Do favors and nice things for other people so that they will feel obligated to you. If people feel obligated to you, they will assist you in achieving your goals and will support you.

Display 5-7
SAMPLE NURSE MANAGER
POSITIVE AFFIRMATIONS

Short-Term Objectives	*Positive Affirmations*
1. By _____ , 19 _____ , I have enrolled in a graduate program.	I am a confident graduate student. I am enthusiastic about completing graduate studies. I am an excellent student.
2. By _____ , 19 _____ , I have a mentor.	I am becoming an outstanding nurse leader.
3. By _____ , 19 _____ , I have completed a management class.	I am an effective manager. I make good management decisions.
4. By _____ , 19 _____ , I have developed a written-down plan to be a nurse manager within two years.	I am the nurse manager of my emergency department. I am a very charismatic nurse leader. I make a difference in nursing.

Never lie or break your word. If you do this even once, people never forget. Once you get a good or bad reputation, it tends to stick. If you have a good reputation, value and protect it. If you have a bad reputation in the organization, you may not be able to overcome it and you may need to go to another organization to accomplish your goals.

Never ask if you can do something if what you want to do is consistent with the organization's values and mission and is legal, ethical, and does not cost too much. If you frequently take action, you will get the reputation for being action-oriented and goal-directed. On the other hand, if you always seek permission, you will be viewed as being hesitant, unsure of yourself, and timid.

Be visible in many different settings. If you are visible, people assume you are accomplishing a lot of things and are very energetic.

Associate with positive, powerful people because their influence will rub off on you. Others will also assume that you are powerful if you associate with successful people, and they will let you do things without questioning you.

Act out conversations on selling your ideas to your boss with a trusted colleague. Your colleague should play your boss so that you can be ready to respond to and overcome objections to your idea and so that you come across as polished and prepared. You can also use this strategy to act out coaching and counseling sessions with difficult employees. By practicing before your session, you will perform better and feel more confident.

Never complain, gripe, or exhibit signs of burn-out as the leader because this behavior is irresponsible and unprofessional for nurse managers. Your job is always to role model the behavior you expect of your staff. If you have irreconcilable differences with your boss or organization, your professional responsibility demands that you resign.

Learn to take calculated risks. If you consider the worst-case scenario, then taking action really involves no risk. Risk stimulates; security and the status quo stifle. Security is associated with boredom, burn-out, monotony, fatigue, and decay. Risks are associated with courage, vision, rewards, power, adventure, enthusiasm, and accomplishments.

Have fun at work through your own personal growth and development. If you are not having fun, find another role or job.

Use personnel selection to assist your unit in actualizing your vision. By selecting a staff that shares your vision, you will be able to actualize it faster.

Always read the professional journals that your boss reads. If you do this, you will be able to anticipate future assignments and will be more in sync with your boss, which can help you to attain your professional goals.

Stay close to all your stakeholders and make their satisfaction your top priority at all times.

Be a mentor to your staff as well as to colleagues from other organizations who approach you. You will only get back from the profession after you put in or make unselfish contributions.

SUMMARY

The future of the profession of nursing depends on the quality and commitment of the current and future nurse managers in health care organizations. The role of the nurse manager will be significantly more influential in the organization in the future, and nurses that desire to meet this kind of a challenge must invest time, energy, and resources in developing themselves to meet this challenge. The future of the profession, quality of patient care outcomes, and viability of health care organizations depend on an adequate number of professional nurses taking on this challenge.

6

Developing
an Executive Image

This chapter presents key issues that have socialized existing nurse executives and compares the role and responsibility of the chief nurse in the present and the future health care organization. It presents a plan for nurse managers to develop an executive image, as well as initiatives to assist existing nurse executives to be successful. The chapter outlines the internal and external stakeholders for the nurse executive and presents some of the pertinent rules of administration to assist them to be more effective and successful in their executive roles. It is also designed to assist aspiring nurse executives to make an informed decision about the nurse executive role appropriate for them.

HISTORICAL SOCIALIZATION OF
NURSE EXECUTIVES

Few of today's nurse executives aspired to the role as young children, adolescents, or new professionals. Traditionally, the nurses who were successful in clinical nursing were singled out by authority figures to become the leaders or managers of nursing units. If head nurses did a good job, they usually went on to head entire nursing departments as directors of nursing. Typically, nurse managers pursued the position of director of nursing only after they received significant encouragement

KEY CHAPTER CONCEPTS

Key Concept #1

A strong desire to be a successful nurse executive is an important prerequisite for becoming a successful nurse executive.

Key Concept #2

A successful nurse executive must earn the trust and respect of a broad range of internal and external stakeholders by being able to communicate with them from their perspective.

Key Concept #3

Effective nurse executives are visionaries, innovators, coaches, facilitators, and exceptional role models.

Key Concept #4

Internal and external stakeholders observe the nurse executive constantly. For an executive, the most important responsibility is to role model the values of the organization and profession every day.

Key Concept #5

Confident and assertive behavior and actions are a requirement for acquiring and maintaining organizational power.

Key Concept #6

Professional appearance is a key component of executive image and communicates how you see yourself and your responsibility to your organization and your profession.

Key Concept #7

Successful nurse executives have advanced skills and education in the business disciplines of financial analysis, marketing, strategic thinking and planning, cost accounting, and systems analysis.

from their peers or superiors. Most directors of nursing learned their role through on-the-job training or after-the-fact education. After-the-fact education means going back to school to obtain an undergraduate or graduate degree after becoming a director of nursing in order to acquire advanced credentials and theoretical skills required in the position.

There are exceptions to this typical scenario, but for the most part this is the way the careers of many directors of nursing progressed. This scenario is changing as a result of the increased number of nurses attending universities for undergraduate and graduate education. However, the typical scenario has determined the perceptions of many people about the past and present role of the nurse executive. It has also influenced the way experienced directors of nursing have been coached and developed and how they have coached, developed, and mentored new nurse executives.

ORGANIZATIONS AND LEADERS OF THE FUTURE

Over the past few decades, the management of organizations has been influenced mainly by the military model. Good managers gave succinct and direct orders, made decisions under fire, and were analytical thinkers and rational decision-makers. Contemporary researchers predict that the leader of the future will be a facilitator, cheerleader, visionary, teacher, and nurturer/mentor (Bennis & Nanus, 1985; Kanter, 1989).

These new leadership characteristics tend to be more feminine in nature than the traits that dominated the military management style. This presents a key opportunity for women and nurses to be effective leaders in their organizations and to acquire the recognition and rewards associated with successful leadership. This new leadership focus is the stimulus for *Key Concept #2.*

In her recent book, *When Giants Learn to Dance,* Kanter proposed that successful companies of the future will need to restructure and rethink operations to achieve the flexibility and focused management required in an environment of constant technological change. Kanter outlined specific shifts in the roles, responsibilities, and nature of organizational power that she predicts will occur in the 1990s. She believes executives will need to focus most of their efforts on juggling their constituencies and consulting with their multiple stakeholders rather than controlling their subordinates. Position in the organization will have less significance and formal power in the future. According to Kanter, executives who can discuss key issues with all their stakeholders in the organization and who seek to gain consensus on what needs to be done will be the successful leaders of the future (Kanter, 1989).

Female leadership models typically rely more on consensus-building and cooperation with others than male leadership models (Helgesen, 1990). The male leadership style is typically more competitive. A female leader's goal is usually more focused on providing a quality outcome, while a male leader's goal is more focused on winning. The female approach to problem-solving is more intuitive; the male approach is more pragmatic and rational. According to Kanter (1989), leaders will need to combine the bias for action of the male leader with the cooperative qualities of the female leader to be effective.

Changes in worker values and the nature of work will demand that managers collaborate with their staff rather than giving orders. Today's workers expect their leaders to challenge them, recognize their accomplishments, and respect them as valuable assets of the organization (Schwartz, 1986). The Japanese style of management and the progression to an information age have shifted American leadership to a more people-oriented focus rather than the industrial or assembly-line management style of the past. This more people-oriented management environment creates opportunities for female leaders because of their socialized focus on relationships.

FUTURE CHALLENGES FOR THE
NURSE EXECUTIVE ROLE

These organizational trends mandate that nurse executives acquire the ability, skill, and commitment to involve their nurse managers and professional staff in all issues affecting patient care delivery and their immediate work units. This means letting go of the need to make most of the decisions. You must be able to allow nurse managers to manage differently on different units and overcome the need to maintain standardization throughout the patient care areas. This means allowing nurse managers to make their own mistakes but being there to support and encourage them. It means being comfortable with taking calculated risks and being able to overcome the by-the-book mentality traditionally seen in many hospitals.

This letting-go process requires a strong positive self-image so that you can delegate management responsibilities and authority to managers and nurses closer to patient care delivery and allow them to make their own decisions and mistakes. Delegation of responsibility to unit-based department directors with twenty-four-hour accountability needs to be accompanied by an adequate amount of authority to match this responsibility. It also means avoiding second-guessing or saying, "I would have done it this way."

Effective nurse leaders are visionaries, facilitators, and exceptional role models. They must develop an ability to influence others through their vision, rather than relying on the formal authority of their position *(Key Concept #3)*. This means learning to negotiate rather than command or direct. In this environment, personality, interpersonal communication skills, and ability to influence through vision will be more important to success as a leader than they were in the bureaucratic organization.

Many organizations and chief executive officers will not readily adopt these new changes. They will be at various stages in the transition from a bureaucratic organization to a decentralized, participative organization. As a nurse executive with a reporting relationship to a leader with more organizational power, you will need to assess where your organization is in this transition and adapt your leadership style to your organization. If the style of your existing or future organization is drastically different from your leadership style, you do not have a good fit. This incongruence will create significant problems for you as an executive. In this case, you should look for an organization and chief executive officer that have a leadership philosophy and values similar to your own to maximize your accomplishments and potential for success.

Two major sources of stress and burn-out for nurse executives are role conflict and role ambiguity (Hardy, 1978). Role conflict is incongruence in the expectations associated with a role. Role ambiguity is a lack of clarity about the changing expectations for a specific role. In the rapidly changing health care environment of the 1990s, the stress created by these two characteristics of the nurse executive role will drastically increase.

Scalzi (1988) studied 124 nurse executives in Los Angeles hospitals and identified their major sources of stress and the coping strategies they used in their role. The four major stresses identified were job overload, quality of care concerns, role conflict, and role ambiguity. Job overload was defined as (1) conflicting expectations from hospital administration and the nursing department, (2) too large a span of control, (3) too many expectations from the job in general, and (4) difficulty managing personal time. The current trends in health care organizations are significantly increasing all these factors for the nurse executive.

PROFILE OF THE NURSE EXECUTIVE

In 1986, Witt and Associates (1987) conducted a survey of nurse executives in hospitals with 250 or more beds to identify the profile of a typical nurse executive. The questionnaire was answered by 377 nurse executives, for a response rate of 26%. Their survey showed:

- Nine percent of nurse executives had the title of associate administrator, 49% were vice-presidents, 15% were assistant administrators, and 26% were directors of nursing.
- The average tenure for nurse executives was 4.8 years.
- The average salary for nurse executives was $56,727.
- The average salary for nurse executives was associated with age, sex, marital status, and education.
- Approximately 50% of nurse executives were eligible for bonuses. The average bonus was 10% of base salary.
- Approximately 50% of nurse executives reported to the president, chief executive officer, or administrator.
- Twenty-three percent of nurse executives had non-patient-care departments such as housekeeping, central supply, pharmacy, and medical library reporting to them.
- Eighty-seven percent of the nurse executives belonged to the American Organization of Nurse Executives (AONE). Less than 10% belonged to the American Management Association or the American College of Healthcare Executives (ACHE).

- Seventy-five percent of nurse executives had at least one Master's degree and 4% had a doctorate degree. Thirty-nine percent of nurse executives had an MSN degree.

The profile for the nurse executive of the future is anticipated to move in the following four directions. First, more graduate programs in nursing will include courses such as finance, accounting, marketing, and strategic planning in their curriculums. In some programs these courses will be offered and taught by professors from the school of business. This is already starting to happen in some programs. This trend will provide the nurse executive with a broader theory base to fulfill the executive role in the organization.

Second, more nurse executives will pursue a Master's degree in business administration. Currently, many nurse leaders are returning for this degree as a second graduate degree so that they can function more effectively. Successful nurse executives need advanced skills and education in financial analysis, marketing, strategic thinking and planning, cost accounting, and systems analysis *(Key Concept #7)*. A Master's degree in business administration will provide them with these skills so that they do not have to acquire them on the job.

Third, more nurse executives will assume the role of chief operating officer (COO) or chief executive officer (CEO) in their organizations. As downsizing occurs, astute CEOs and governing boards are realizing that successful nurse executives can manage nonnursing departments very effectively. Generic executives without a clinical or nursing background usually cannot manage nursing departments successfully in the long run. When top-level management positions need to be downsized, the effective nurse executive has a competitive edge over the generic executive. This will increase the feeling of job overload for some nurse executives, as expressed in Scalzi's research. However, the dynamic nurse executive will see this role as a key opportunity to make significant changes on behalf of nursing and the delivery of quality patient care. By having responsibility for day-to-day operations of the entire organization, the nurse executive can identify and eliminate the inefficiencies that typically occur at the boundaries between the clinical, ancillary, and support departments. This is a more effective way of responding to needed expense reductions than reducing nursing hours or diluting the professional staffing mix.

This trend will also increase the feeling of role ambiguity and role conflict for many nurse executives. Some nurse executives will rise to the challenge, while others will not. Successful nurse executives will make the transition from a nurse who happens to be an executive to an executive who happens to be a nurse. Nurse leaders who focus exclusively on managing clinical nursing issues will be limited in their contributions because of their narrow perspective of the patient care delivery process.

Fourth, more nurse executives will return for their doctorate degrees to be more competitive in university-based organizations, to establish themselves as legitimate leaders in the health care industry, and to fulfill their own professional goals. In an environment in which a Master's degree is a minimum standard for executives, a doctorate provides a competitive edge.

This puts additional stress on many nurse executives as they attempt to balance their executive role with the role of a student. Some will temporarily drop out of the workforce to complete this degree. Nurse executives will feel the pressure on their personal commitments and lifestyle. Some people who really want to complete their doctorate but who do not feel that they can make the commitment for professional or personal reasons will feel frustrated and resentful. Others will pay the price of strained family and professional relationships to complete their postgraduate studies.

This educational trend will also have a dramatic effect on the relationships between nursing, CEOs, and physicians. It will elevate nursing's position in the organization, but will create tensions between competent and confident nurse executives and insecure administrators and physicians. The confident nurse executive must anticipate and prepare for a potential backlash from these internal stakeholders who may feel threatened but nevertheless have significant influence in the organization.

It may also widen the gap between the clinical nurse and the nurse executive if staff nurses do not also seek advanced education. If clinical nurses do not pursue Bachelor's and graduate degrees, the nurse executive will need to be able to maintain meaningful dialogue with them despite a significant difference in perspective resulting from a wide variation in education levels and daily responsibilities.

On the other hand, this is a key opportunity for nurse executives to encourage their nurses to pursue advanced education and to insist on certain minimum levels of education for specific roles. Therefore, this trend toward higher education has the potential to raise the standard of professionalism throughout the organization.

ASSESSING YOUR EXECUTIVE READINESS

It is important to be in touch with the perceptions of nurse executives and to understand the future trends for the role so that you can make an educated decision about the best role for you. Before you make the commitment of time and energy, and pursue advanced education, you need to understand all aspects of the role to make the best decision for your career.

A strong desire to be a successful nurse executive is the most important prerequisite for becoming a successful nurse executive *(Key Concept #1)*. To help you decide if you are ready to make the commitment to a nurse executive role, complete the short readiness questionnaire (Display 6-1). The questionnaire is by no means scientific, but it can help you decide if you are willing and ready to undertake some of the actions and pay some of the prices that are necessary to be a success in the role. If you answered "no" to four or more of these questions, you have some additional work and contemplation to do before you set a goal to become a nurse executive.

NEW ROLE, RESPONSIBILITIES, AND EXPECTATIONS

As a nurse executive, you will experience the expectations, responsibilities, and rewards of an executive in the business world. You will need to become acutely in tune with the political arena of your organization. Understand who has the informal and formal power, the historical issues that drive current organizational decision-making, and the key timing issues for your organization. Develop the ability to always be positive when you are in public, be able to role model the organization's values all of the time, develop your desired vision for your organization, be a time-management expert, and be comfortable taking calculated risks to move your organization toward your desired vision.

Display 6-1
NURSE EXECUTIVE
READINESS QUESTIONNAIRE

	Yes	*No*

1. I have a strong desire to lead nurses through an executive role.

2. I am prepared and willing to commit up to sixty hours per week to be successful.

3. I am prepared to pay whatever price I need to pay to obtain a graduate degree.

4. I believe I can be a successful nurse executive.

5. I am comfortable making difficult and unpopular decisions to provide quality patient care in new and different ways.

6. I have a solid support system outside my work environment.

7. I believe I can accomplish anything I set my mind to.

8. I do not require recognition by others to know I have done a good job and to be satisfied with my accomplishments.

9. Being respected by my employees is more important for me than being liked by them.

10. I am prepared emotionally and economically to be fired at any time as a nurse executive.

Display 6-1 *(continued)*
NURSE EXECUTIVE
READINESS QUESTIONNAIRE

	Yes	*No*

11. I am committed to reading at least three professional journals per week to keep myself current on industry issues.

12. I set and write down annual goals.

13. I am comfortable in an ambiguous environment in which the rules of the game change daily.

14. I can alter my communication style to fit my audience without feeling that I am compromising myself.

As a successful nurse executive, you will need to learn to be competitive, analytical, unemotional, and an aggressive team player in a male-dominated corporate culture. You should be able to incorporate these characteristics into your personality and be comfortable with possessing these characteristics. In addition to these male characteristics, you should be able to incorporate into your leadership style the female behaviors of cooperation, intuitive-rational problem-solving techniques, empathy, collaboration, and empowerment of others.

According to Bennis and Nanus (1985), contemporary leaders need to develop their skills in four major areas: the ability to develop a vision for their organization; the ability to communicate that vision to their stakeholders; the ability to establish trust in their stakeholders; and the ability to maintain a strong, positive self-image. The development of a strong, positive self-image is the most important skill because it drives the other three abilities. You cannot develop an organizational vision, communicate that vision, or instill trust in people if you do not have a positive, confident professional self-image. Your self-image is a powerful influence on the performance and achievements of your professional staff.

According to Stew Leonard, owner of the very successful Stew Leonard's Dairy, "Morale comes down from the sky like rain. If you're the boss and you're feeling lousy—watch out—you're like the plague going around. If I wake up in a terrible mood, I don't go to the store, I work at home. I don't want to bring any of my people down" (Olsen, 1988). It is crucial to adopt this kind of thinking and action if you are a nurse executive. The role has the responsibility always to be positive and to be an effective role model for your staff. This may require either staying away from your staff or managers when you are not feeling positive or doing an exceptional job of "acting" positive. As a nurse executive, you have the responsibility always to rise to this challenge because your internal and external stakeholders observe you constantly. As an executive, your most important responsibility is to role model the values of your organization and your profession every day *(Key Concept #4)*.

ASSESSING AND DEVELOPING YOUR LEADERSHIP STYLE

Leadership in the 1990s is moving toward a more charismatic, take-charge role. The leader of the future will be more visible and out in front, leading the team by example. Effective leaders are expected to be visionaries. Visionaries inspire their staff to believe in and buy into their goals for the organization and to work hard together to achieve those goals.

If your leadership style is more passive or autocratic in nature, it is possible to change it to enable you to fit this changing environment. The following steps can help you to move your leadership style toward a more visionary style.

Step One:
Assess Your Current Leadership Style

You can assess your leadership style by asking for feedback from a trusted peer, colleague, or subordinate. This request can be threatening for subordinates; however, it can be less threatening if you design a confidential and directed feedback form for them to fill out.

A directed feedback form is a questionnaire that includes questions about the specific traits you want feedback on, rather than asking open-ended questions such as "Please evaluate my leadership style." An example of a directed feedback question is:

	Always				*Never*
My supervisor is approachable and available to me when I have a problem.	5	4	3	2	1

Nurse managers with positive self-images are usually comfortable providing their boss with constructive feedback. Requesting and receiving this feedback requires a positive, strong self-image because you may receive feedback that you do not expect or are not prepared for. Feedback is a person's perception of you, how they see you based on who they are. Their perceptions should never be considered right or wrong, good or bad. A person's perceptions are real for them and for you because they determine how that person relates to you. A person's perceptions of you tell you the impact you have on them, and this knowledge can help you to identify ways to become more effective in relating to them and getting the results you really desire.

If you do not have a strong, positive self-image, you may make excuses for other people's perceptions of you or may not make attempts to receive feedback. These behaviors are a clue that you need to work on improving your self-image so that you do not avoid feedback or interpret it negatively. Become confident enough in yourself to view constructive feedback as a tool to assist you in modifying your behavior and individualizing your communication with others in order to be more effective and successful in the future.

Step Two:
Assess the Leadership Style Your
Major Stakeholders Respond to Best

You can find out what style of leadership your stakeholders respond to by asking them the following questions: What can I do as a leader to make you more successful? Do you appreciate specific direction on what needs to be done and how to do it or do you like to understand the goal and then be left alone?

It is wrong to assume that everyone likes to be treated and led the same way or the way you do. People evaluate your leadership ability based on how well you relate to them and respond to their individual needs. They evaluate your effectiveness based on how well you meet their needs rather than how well you meet the organization's goals or your own goals.

Step Three:
Adapt Your Leadership Style to
Your Stakeholders

After assessing your existing leadership style and your stakeholders' individual needs and preferences for leadership, you can take steps to adapt your style to be more effective with each of your stakeholders. Periodically request feedback on how close you are approximating their leadership preferences to determine your progress. These actions will not be seen as a weakness by your stakeholders. They will feel very good that you care enough about them to alter your style to meet their individual needs. People who do not continually develop themselves as leaders will not be successful in their organizations in the long run.

DEVELOPING AN EXECUTIVE SELF-IMAGE

People's common expectations for an executive drive their assessment of whether or not a person is acting like an executive. When you look like an executive, you will be treated like one. Common expectations or assumptions about executives include:

- Executives are knowledgeable.
- Executives are self-controlled.
- Executives are confident and poised.
- Executives have a specific physical appearance:
    - They appear healthy and trim.
    - They have a solid presence that communicates they are in control.
    - They do not wear trendy business attire.
    - They always appear neat and well-groomed.
    - Their shoes always appear polished.
- Executives appear able to handle any and all difficult situations.
- Executives appear to handle stress well.

- Executives work long hours.
- Executives have completed graduate education.
- Executives communicate well verbally and in writing.
- Executives are decisive.
- Executives get things done.
- Executives are energetic and enthusiastic.

Any and all strategies for developing the self-image of a nurse executive need to focus on developing these traits and characteristics in your daily routine and way of presenting yourself. If you have philosophical problems with developing any of these traits or characteristics, you will have difficulty developing an executive self-image and may not be treated like an executive. People who desire to develop the self-image of an executive often feel funny or awkward when they first decide to change their image. This is a normal feeling that goes away once you have internalized the role.

The overall process to assist you in transforming your self-image from nurse practitioner to executive or from nurse manager to nurse executive follows. The process includes developing a strong desire for the role, setting a professional goal to be a nurse executive, developing short-term objectives to get to this professional goal, developing and repeating positive affirmations, and visualizing yourself as an executive.

Step One:
Take Responsibility for Your
Professional Self

The first step in developing an executive self-image is to have a strong desire to become a nurse executive and to make a conscious decision to pay the price of attaining your goal. All future steps require that you make this decision.

There are many nurse executives in the industry who were pushed into the role by bosses, colleagues, significant others, or instructors, but who never really decided to pay the price required to be successful. Many of these nurse executives are currently disenchanted, frustrated, and ineffective in their role because they never really desired the role. If you are one of these nurse executives, you need to reassess your priorities. Fill out the readiness questionnaire included in this chapter (Display 6-1, pp. 152–153) to determine whether you want to stay in the role or look for a different role that better meets your personal and professional priorities. If you are not enjoying the role, you should get out of it as soon as possible. You are not a failure if this is how you feel. You are simply facing the fact that you do not enjoy the role and realize that you owe it to yourself to be happy and content in your professional life.

Step Two:
Define Your Executive Goal

If you have made the decision to commit yourself to becoming a nurse executive, set a two-year goal for the specific role you desire. Decide exactly what type of organization you want to be a nurse executive in. Decide whether you want to be a director of nursing, vice-president for nursing, vice-president for patient care services, chief operating officer, corporate vice-president for nursing, or the president of your own consulting firm. These are all nurse executive roles with very different implications and responsibilities.

Write your specific professional goal down on paper using the guidelines outlined in previous chapters. The goal has to be written in the present tense, with a specific deadline for its accomplishment. A sample professional goal for a nurse executive would be: *By_____ , 19___ , I am the vice-president for nursing at a two-hundred-bed community hospital in Southern California.*

Step Three:
Executive Self-Assessment

Complete an assessment of your current professional situation in order to identify the major areas on which you need to focus to attain your nurse executive role in the next two years. A nurse executive self-assessment appears in Display 6-2.

Step Four:
Develop Short-Term Objectives for
Your Executive Role

After completing your executive assessment, develop three short-term objectives that can be accomplished within one year that respond to the differences between your current self-image and the self-image of a nurse executive.

(text continues on page 162)

Display 6-2
NURSE EXECUTIVE SELF-ASSESSMENT

Executive Characteristics	Your Current Self-Image	Nurse Executive Self-Image
Graduate education		Master's degree
Knowledge of nursing issues, leadership issues, hospital financial issues, reimbursement issues, JCAHO issues, licensing issues, medical staff issues, governing body issues, health care industry issues, and legal issues		In-depth and up-to-date knowledge in all these areas
Business attire		Nontrendy business suits and dresses; closed-toe pumps; no low-cut necklines; no see-through tops
Classic jewelry		No dangling earrings; classic gold or silver pieces; no plastic beads
Briefcase		Black, brown, or burgundy leather briefcase
Purse		Small and organized; when carrying a purse and briefcase, purse needs to fit inside of briefcase

(continued)

Display 6-2 *(continued)*
NURSE EXECUTIVE SELF-ASSESSMENT

Executive Characteristics	*Your Current Self-Image*	*Nurse Executive Self-Image*
Political savvy		Good understanding of who to say what to and when. Good timing; knowledge of who has the informal power and how to make the boss look good
Self-control		Never cry or appear tired or overwhelmed in public; never get so angry that you lose your control and composure
Time-management skills		Learn how to get the important things done before your deadlines; learn to do more than one thing at a time
Need for recognition of accomplishments		None; you get your satisfaction from completing projects and observing your staff succeed
Ability to sell ideas		Excellent selling skills to get your ideas approved by your boss

Display 6-2 *(continued)*
NURSE EXECUTIVE SELF-ASSESSMENT

Executive Characteristics	*Your Current Self-Image*	*Nurse Executive Self-Image*
Vision		Can see very clearly in your mind how you would like nursing to function, look, and perform in the future
Executive self-image		See yourself as confident, decisive, tough, and able to handle anything that comes your way
Assertive communication		Able to give and receive constructive feedback in a direct, nondefensive manner; able to be direct in very political situations
Response to high-risk environment		Emotionally and economically prepared to be fired at any time
Response to ambiguous environment		Love change

Display 6-3
SHORT-TERM EXECUTIVE OBJECTIVES

1. By _____ , 19 _____ ,
   I am knowledgeable about who has the formal and informal
   power in my organization.

2. By _____ , 19 _____ ,
   I look like a nurse executive.

3. By _____ , 19 _____ ,
   I am enrolled in a doctorate program.

4. By _____ , 19 _____ ,
   I have learned the principles of effective selling.

5. By _____ , 19 _____ ,
   I know how to develop a marketing plan for a clinical service.

6. By _____ , 19 _____ ,
   I know how to develop a business plan.

7. By _____ , 19 _____ ,
   I have a professional article accepted for publication.

Examples of some short-term objectives that you can use if you are a nurse manager setting a goal to become a nurse executive are given in Display 6-3.

Take action today to accomplish one of your short-term objectives. Actions you could take include investigating graduate education programs in your area, going shopping to purchase a new suit, going to a beauty salon to have your hair done in a style more appropriate for an executive, getting an executive make-over to assist in choosing appropriate clothes and makeup, or subscribing to the *Journal of Nursing Administration*, *Modern Healthcare*, or *Hospitals* magazine to start keeping informed on industry and leadership issues.

Step Five:
Program Yourself for Your
Executive Role

Find or create a picture of yourself as an executive and put it on your refrigerator so that you can daily reprogram your self-image as an executive. Make sure the picture depicts exactly the way you want to be perceived by others and includes the specific type of business attire and image that communicates your desired executive role.

There are many different messages you can communicate through your business attire and accessories. Make a decision whether you want to come across as scholarly, conservative, flamboyant, moderate, preppy, maternal, or businesslike. After you have defined your executive image, determine the specific clothes and accessories that will help you to communicate that specific executive image.

Develop positive affirmations for each short-term objective based on the guidelines covered in Chapter Three and repeat these affirmations daily. Display 6-4 outlines positive affirmations that you could use to accomplish specific short-term objectives.

POWER AND THE NURSE EXECUTIVE ROLE

Power is the energy required to initiate and sustain action to translate all intentions into reality (Bennis & Nanus, 1985). Effective leaders need power to actualize their organizational visions. Leaders need strong, positive self-images to develop the personal power to lead their people and organizations effectively in an ambiguous and rapidly changing environment.

Leaders with positive self-images rarely have to rely on criticism or sanctions to get others to perform well. Leaders with positive self-images portray confidence in their own abilities and the abilities of their employees. This confidence makes employees rise to and perform up to the expectations of their leaders.

When you empower others to achieve their goals as well as the organization's goals, you acquire the ability to translate your intentions into reality. Your organization can be successful when you communicate your desired vision for the organization, empower your workforce, and trust your employees to attain your vision for the organization.

Display 6-4
SAMPLE NURSE EXECUTIVE
POSITIVE AFFIRMATIONS

Short-Term Objectives	*Positive Affirmations*
1. By _____ , 19 ____ , I am knowledgeable about the formal and informal power in my organization.	I feel confident about my skill and ability to communicate with many people outside my department.
	I am excited about the ability to work with others to get to my goals and help them get to their goals.
2. By _____ , 19 ____ , I have the appearance of a nurse executive.	I feel confident and poised in my executive role.
	I am decisive and confident in my executive decisions.
	I feel comfortable with my executive appearance.
3. By _____ , 19 ____ , I am enrolled in a doctorate program.	I am challenged by my studies as a doctoral student.

A nurse executive needs to acquire a broader base of power than a nurse manager to be able to get things done in the political environment of the executive. In this environment, the way to be successful is to accomplish your goals while assisting your stakeholders to accomplish their goals. This becomes a major challenge because of the large number of stakeholders the nurse executive has. Assertive communication skills and actions are needed to influence these multiple stakeholders to accomplish goals.

As a nurse executive, your stakeholders within the organization include your boss, patients and their families, physicians, nurses, administrative peers, department directors, and nurse managers. Stakeholders outside the organization that significantly influence nurse executives include regulatory agencies, accreditation agencies, the community, future patients, the media, lobbyists, professional organizations, existing and future labor pool, other health care providers, competitors, the legal system, philanthropists, the educational system, and your colleagues. To be truly effective as a nurse executive, you must be able to influence all these stakeholders by earning their respect and trust so that they will support you in accomplishing your desired vision for the organization.

Benziger (1985) identified a number of ways women typically respond to people they do not like but who can significantly assist or interfere with their power base in an organization. Women often respond to people they do not like by avoiding them. This is because many women were socialized as young girls to stop playing with children they did not like or that did not play by the rules. Boys, on the other hand, were typically more involved in team sports and learned that the goal was to win the game even if there were children on the team whom they did not like.

Such avoidance behavior decreases your power base and does not allow you to influence anyone. Women often do not acknowledge that they dislike other people and typically describe these relationships as "personality conflicts." They also may have difficulty being direct about their negative feelings toward other women. They may tell other people that they have problems with a particular person rather than directing those negative feelings toward that person. Women have the capability to develop positive relationships with people they do not like but many choose not to.

Many men have traditionally learned through their participation in team sports that if you want to be chosen the leader, you need to earn the trust and respect of people you like as well as those you dislike. These men have learned that winning takes precedence over any and all personal feelings about people on the team.

The most appropriate and effective way to respond to people you do not particularly like is to be assertive. Assertive communication and behavior demonstrate that you recognize and respect people for who they are and expect them to treat you in a similar manner. Assertive behavior and communication patterns are a prerequisite for influencing others and increasing your power in the organization to accomplish the organization's goals.

STRATEGIES TO INCREASE YOUR ORGANIZATIONAL AND PERSONAL POWER

Organizational power is the power that exists within organizations to accomplish their goals. Formal organizational power is typically described by the organizational chart, which depicts the level of formal power people have as a function of their role. Organizational power also includes informal power, or the personal power that people in the organization possess irrespective of their formal role or position.

According to the Zero Sum theory, power in an organization is conceptualized as a fixed commodity. Therefore, if one person's power base is increased in an organization, there is a resulting decrease in power for others.

Organizations also have varying levels of movement or exchange of power based on whether they are dynamic or stable organizations. Dynamic organizations are constantly changing in response to their external environment, and this change results in movement of power from one role to another and from one department to another. Stable or static organizations, which experience less change in response to their environment, tend to maintain power in the same roles and departments.

In dynamic organizations, power is constantly up for grabs for people and groups that are thriving, innovating, and actively responding to change. The people or groups within the organization that desire to maintain the status quo tend to lose ground in this environment.

As a nurse executive responsible for the largest group of health care professionals in the organization, you need to respond constantly to your internal and external environment to maintain and increase your share of organizational power. This responsibility to acquire maximum organizational power is not for your own personal gain or use but is important to represent your patients, physicians, and nurses adequately. It is not something you can abdicate by being low-key, polite, accommodating, or compliant. If you respond in any of these ways, you will lose organizational power and your nursing staff, physicians, and patients will suffer.

As a nurse executive, you have a responsibility to determine what needs to be done, within what timeframe things need to happen, and who the right people are to present your ideas to in your organization. This is important for maintaining an adequate share of organizational power so that you can actualize your vision for your staff and patients.

Maintaining your share of power is something you must consider a major responsibility if you plan to make the necessary organizational changes demanded by professional nurses, the profession, and the public.

Nurse executives have the responsibility actively to seek out maximum organizational power to be able to deal effectively and successfully with the problems that need to be solved in health care organizations. Such problems include:

1. Eliminating salary compression problems within the nursing wage and salary structure.
2. Reducing the level of tension and conflict between nurses and physicians in your organization. The leading source of stress for clinical nurses in most acute care facilities is poor communication and interpersonal relationships with physicians.
3. Enhancing the image of professional nurses in your organization.
4. Empowering professional nurses and nurse managers in your organization to be able to make decisions about patient care delivery and their immediate work group and work unit.
5. Redesigning hospital operations to enhance patient care delivery and reduce stakeholder frustration.
6. Enhancing the quality and level of care and service for patients, physicians, and patients' families.
7. Retaining qualified and caring professional nurses.

There are a number of strategies to enhance your organizational power to accomplish your goals for your stakeholders. For example, *a.* learn to get tough. This means being able to endure difficult situations without quitting or becoming emotional in public situations. A public situation is any situation in which you are with one of your stakeholders. Remember, your stakeholders include your patients, staff, peers, boss, and physicians.

b. Learn to speak the language of the power brokers in your organization. In hospitals this means learning the quantifiable language of the chief financial officer and the administrator. When you have mastered that language, you need to be able to talk with all your major stakeholders in the language that is meaningful to them. By speaking their language, you make them comfortable and do not intimidate them, and they identify with you and trust you. When you rely on administrative jargon to communicate with physicians, nurses, and patients, you alienate them and widen the gap between your role and theirs.

An example of a typical communication gap is when a nurse executive talks "nurse talk" to an administrator who only talks and understands quantifiable or bottom-line terms. These conversations are typically very frustrating for both parties and usually little gets accomplished.

Talking "nurse talk" makes nonnurses uncomfortable and inhibits your ability to make your point and get what you want. Once you begin speaking in the language of each one of your stakeholders, you experience fewer frustrations and get what you want because your stakeholders are comfortable with you and understand what you want.

This strategy includes identifying and using or avoiding key words that turn your stakeholders off or on. When you learn to use the words that are important to them and eliminate the use of words that make them uncomfortable, you will see dramatic results in your effectiveness. Display 6-5 lists a number of words and phrases to use or avoid with your various stakeholders.

c. Align your priorities with the priorities of your boss and the top leader in your organization. Learn to articulate your goals and ideas in terms of their priorities and language to ensure that those priorities get the proper attention, resources, and timely approval.

d. Develop strong working relationships with key power brokers in your organization irrespective of who they report to. You must develop personal influence with the informal leaders throughout your organization to be truly effective and to accomplish your goals.

Develop strong, assertive communication skills and actions. This means being able to be direct with people throughout the organization, including your peers and your boss. Be able to confront peers or subordinates who hope you will fail or you will be victimized by them. Direct communication allows you to accomplish things in a much shorter timeframe because you cut out much of the game playing.

e. Become an expert in something that is important to your organization and its leaders. You can find out what is important to the organization by reading the long-range plan for your organization,

**Display 6-5
WORDS AND PHRASES TO USE
OR AVOID WITH STAKEHOLDERS**

Stakeholder	Words and Phrases to Avoid	Words and Phrases to Use
Care givers	Cost-containment Outcomes Accountability	Quality Acuity
Chief financial officers	Quality of care Prospective payment	Cost-effective Reductions Profitability Revenue enhancement
Chief executive officers	Primary Care Collaborative practice All RN staff	Quality at a lower cost Patient satisfaction Physician satisfaction Profitability
Physicians	DRGs Utilization review Preauthorization Liability	Quality of care Preferential treatment Patient satisfaction

reading what your boss reads, and observing your boss very carefully. Pay close attention to key words or phrases your boss uses and incorporate those words and phrases into your vocabulary. This will communicate to your boss that you are on the same wavelength and in full support of the direction he or she has set.

Always assume a proactive, "I can do it" attitude. When faced with additional responsibilities, work, or projects, always be prepared to say "I can do it" in a very positive, cheerful way. Worry about how you will do it at a later time in the privacy of your office. Powerful people in an organization always come across as very enthusiastic, flexible, and courageous. You do not have to possess all these traits in reality, you just have to create the illusion that you possess them by appearing to be prepared and unshaken by anything.

f. Assume power and authority by doing things that are consistent with the organization's goals and mission for the future. Never ask permission to do things that fit into this category because you will come across as timid and unsure of yourself. When you ask permission, you put additional stress on your boss to assume responsibility for your actions. Take responsibility for your own actions by just doing them. This strategy involves a certain amount of risk-taking, but you only accomplish great things when you take calculated risks.

To avoid taking unnecessary risks, always define the worst-case scenario of your actions. If you are willing to accept this scenario because your idea is so great, you really are not taking any risk. If you cannot accept the worst-case scenario, modify your idea until you can accept the worst-case scenario.

g. Always make your boss look good and publicly give credit to him or her for all your accomplishments. This strategy will ensure your success in the organization, and your boss in turn will give you more freedom, latitude, and margin for error. On the other hand, if you or your performance are a threat to your boss, your days with the organization will be numbered.

Leaders are perpetual learners. They are constantly reading books and journals, attending seminars, continuing their formal education, networking with colleagues to exchange ideas, and learning from their past experiences. Engaging in these activities requires a significant commitment of time, energy, and resources. Managers who aspire to be nurse executives but are not willing to make their career a significant part of their life, to take work home, or to compromise their family or personal lives will not be successful.

EXECUTIVE COMMUNICATION

Pondy (1978) describes leadership as changing employee behavior to accomplish organizational goals and giving meaning to the work people do. Language skills are crucial for leaders because they allow them to communicate their organizational visions. Leaders affect individual behavior when they can speak the language of all of their stakeholders and can communicate meaningfully with them.

Hospitals consist of many specialized groups of stakeholders, each with their own language. Nurses, physicians, patients, and administrators all speak different languages. The successful nurse executive must learn how to relate to and speak with all of these key stakeholders in the language they each understand and identify with. An effective leader speaks in the language of the audience rather than in the language that represents the leader.

As a successful nurse executive you must be comfortable speaking the language of your nurses, physicians, peers, patients and their families, the media, regulatory agencies, the financial department, the marketing department, the legal profession, and your boss. The importance of effective communication is documented by Henry and LeClair (1987), who report that three fourths of a nurse executive's day is spent talking with others.

THE HEALTHY EXECUTIVE

It is important for successful executives to convey an image of being healthy and fit. This is especially true for health care executives. According to a 1983 study by Pelletier at the University of California in San Francisco, healthy executives shared the following beliefs and attitudes about their performance and role:

1. Healthy executives see deregulation, increased competition, and rapid change as a challenge rather than as a threat.
2. Healthy executives get involved by being committed to trying new things.
3. Healthy executives have a sense that they "make a difference" in the changing environment.
4. Healthy executives believe that they are a part of the team and involve everyone in that team effort.
5. Healthy executives take care of themselves physically and emotionally so that they can accomplish all of the above challenges.

You can become a healthy executive by exercising for one hour at least three to five times per week. The challenges and stress of the executive mandate that you be healthy and energetic from a physical and emotional perspective. Exercising allows you to stay physically fit, maintain your endurance, and reduce your frustrations with issues and problems you are confronted with on a daily basis. Routine exercise allows you to get rid of anger or frustration so that you do not carry it around with you. One hour of vigorous activity that results in an increase in heart rate can help you let go of all anger and frustration. Exercise allows you start every day as a new day, without carrying negative issues from one day to the next. If you do not engage in regular exercise, you will not be able consistently to work fifty- to sixty-hour weeks and deal with ongoing crisis situations and changes occurring in your executive role.

MENTORING: THE SOCIALIZATION OF EXECUTIVES

Mentoring is a vehicle for socializing nurse leaders to become politically savvy and personally powerful in their roles. Keep in mind that your behavior and actions are a reflection of your thoughts and beliefs about yourself; therefore, you must have a strong, positive self-image to promote professional growth in the people you are mentoring.

Brockner (1988) reported that social support can make a significant difference in the career achievement of nurses and identified the three major types of support needed by a protégé:

1. Practical support, which includes help and advice on household management, family, and child care issues in relation to the executive role.
2. Emotional support, which includes advice, empathy, and encouragement for one's professional career in relation to one's personal life.
3. Direct support, which involves a variety of activities that help the person to advance in her or his career. This type of support includes introducing the protégé to key people for career advancement, resume writing, and advice on the timing of career moves.

Puetz outlined the benefits of the mentor relationship on the advancement of professionals in their nursing careers (Puetz, 1983). Those benefits include referrals to other professionals, which can provide linkages to information, people, and career opportunities; feedback which can help you evaluate your ideas, performance, and perceptions; career counseling which can assist you with issues including education, politics, timing, and positioning; and access to a role model, which can help you attain your professional goals. Greene and Organ (1973) described the three dimensions of a role that affect job satisfaction: role accuracy, role clarity, and role consensus. A mentor can act as a socializing agent by describing these dimensions for the nurse executive protégé, outlining the variations among facilities, and teaching the protégé how to identify a good fit with the various corporate cultures and organizations.

To acquire the benefits of a mentor relationship, approach a nurse executive you respect and admire in your organization or another organization and ask her or him to help you attain your executive goal. Most nurse executives are flattered when a nurse manager or clinical nurse asks them for professional career counseling or an ongoing mentoring relationship. Your request communicates that they have done something memorable to elicit your admiration and they are usually very happy to give you advice on a one-time or ongoing basis.

After you have established a mentor relationship with a successful nurse executive, be willing to ask for open and honest feedback without becoming defensive. This is one of the best ways to improve your current performance and become the successful executive you want to be.

As a nurse executive, you must project an image of authority, competence, and success. Your attire must be appropriate for your figure, audience, geographic location, and occasion. Stereotypes or assumptions concerning female executives you may need to overcome include:

1. She is more interested in family and personal commitments than in a responsible, long-term career.
2. She is emotional and weak in difficult situations.
3. She is an immature girl.
4. She is naive.
5. She is dependent.
6. She is a sex object.

These stereotypes usually are not discussed openly or covered in any college or university course, but you must acknowledge that they may be underlying assumptions some corporate leaders attribute to women executives. You can learn effective strategies to counteract these typical assumptions through your association and training with an experienced mentor. Your mentor must be willing to share firsthand experiences and strategies with you so that you do not have to learn these lessons by experiencing them yourself. In most cases, your mentor's most valuable lessons have been learned from painful and traumatic experiences, which require a certain level of maturity and self-confidence to share with you. These painful experiences were most likely situations in which your mentor did not perform effectively and felt vulnerable. Here again, a mentor must have a strong, positive self-image to be able to share losses and experiences in which the mentor was not at her or his best for the purpose of assisting you to be successful in these same situations.

A mentor that has a poor or negative self-image and little self-confidence can be a very poor influence and have a detrimental effect on you as a new nurse executive. You will tend to take on the negative and skeptical characteristics of your mentor and mirror your mentor's leadership style. A mentor with a poor self-image may not be able to share painful experiences and may desire on an unconscious level for you to learn the difficult political lessons by experience. The lack of strong, positive role models, leaders, and mentors in nursing is a major reason the profession has not been able to make the transition to a mature profession.

STRATEGIES FOR BECOMING AN EXCELLENT NURSE EXECUTIVE

Multimillionaire H. L. Hunt believed that successful people need to accomplish only two things. First, they need to have a clear idea of exactly what they want to accomplish. Second, they must resolve to pay the price of getting to their goal.

If you have made the decision and commitment to be a successful nurse executive, typically you will need to pay a significant price to be successful. To minimize this price would be to mislead you. If you are committed to being an excellent nurse executive, you will also realize that your job is more secure and that your financial rewards significantly exceed those of the majority of people who are satisfied with just doing their job. According to Tracy (1986), the truly excellent leaders in their respective fields are never out of work despite fluctuations in the economy and always make significantly larger salaries than their mediocre counterparts. Adopt the philosophy that you are not just there to make a living, but there to make a difference.

A number of strategies for becoming an excellent executive have been documented by research in the field, world leaders, books, tapes, and personal experiences. For example, make a personal decision and commitment to excellence or to being the best nurse executive you possibly can be. This strategy requires that you make a conscious decision to go the extra mile and pay the price to be outstanding in your field. You will pay a greater personal and professional price to attain the goal of excellence than the average executive, but you will also receive benefits and rewards that far surpass those of the average executive.

A good rule of thumb is that you only get out of a situation to the degree that you have contributed and only after you have contributed. Some of the specific prices paid and benefits reaped for excellence are listed in Display 6-6. Excellence is a journey rather than an outcome. You never really get there; the excitement and benefits of excellence result from moving closer to the target.

Develop a sense of perseverance and never give up on your goal to be a nurse executive. Perseverance is a measure of your confidence in yourself and your abilities. Persistence is a key word for leaders. Self-confidence is driven by your self-image or the picture you have of yourself. Figure 6-1 (p. 177) outlines the self-image model and emphasizes the importance of perseverance in a commitment to excellence.

Learn to take time to reflect on your successes and maintain an attitude of gratitude. It is easy to focus on the negative things that happen to you and that you have had to overcome. By periodically writing down all of the things you are grateful for, you will be better able to put your career progress into perspective.

The executive gets blamed for everything that goes wrong and rarely gets recognition for the things that go right. You can cope with the outcomes that fall short of your expectations by following these simple guidelines:

1. Acknowledge that things did not work out the way you planned but do not spend time blaming yourself or anyone else.

Display 6-6
PRICES AND BENEFITS OF EXCELLENCE

Price	Benefits
Need to work long hours	Professional respect from colleagues and the industry
Need constantly to improve skills and talents	High level of self-confidence
Need to manage physical self	Increased quality of life
Need to take total responsibility for self	Excellent salary
Need to take calculated risks	Recognition
Need to overcome all fears	Opportunities to advance profession and patient care delivery
Need to focus on the needs and wants of all stakeholders	An increase in organizational and personal power
Can never blame, make excuses, or respond to others defensively	High self-esteem, self-satisfaction, and peace of mind

2. Acknowledge that you survived the incident and that the consequences or outcomes could have been much worse than they actually were.
3. Take any action you feel is necessary to rectify or minimize the problems that occurred as a result of the situation.
4. Identify at least five things you learned as a result of the incident and write them down on a sheet of paper.
5. Set a new goal for yourself in your executive role.

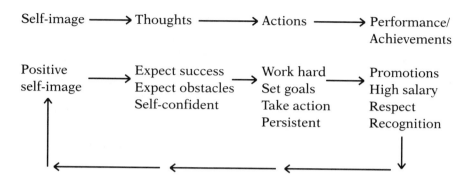

Figure 6-1. Self-Image Model

Stop thinking of your job as work. It is your career and a part of your identity. When people ask you what you do, say you are a nurse executive, rather than saying you are a nurse, a mother, or a wife.

Work to overcome your need to be and act "nice." Replace that thinking and behavior with assertive behavior and a strong desire to be respected for your contributions.

Start taking care of yourself emotionally and economically. Get your own personal checking and savings account and charge cards if you do not already have them. You never know when you might need to establish your own financial track record, and it is better not to have to do it in a crisis situation.

Move from a focus on details to a focus on the big picture and from a short-term perspective to a long-term perspective.

Learn how to create the illusion of being perfect without being a perfectionist. Creating this illusion communicates that you have your act together and are a responsible professional. Being a perfectionist results in rigid behavior and frustration for you and the people you interact with. Perfectionists are not enjoyable people to be around.

Learn how to say no without feeling guilty or being aggressive.

Learn to delegate responsibility, authority, and accountability to others. This requires a significant amount of confidence and trust in yourself as well as others. When you delegate to others, you reduce your level of frustration and communicate that you trust others. This strengthens the bond between you, and you will acquire increased personal power as a result of entrusting power to others.

Learn to act as though you are in control when difficult situations arise, even when you do not know what you are going to do. When faced with a difficult situation, take a couple of deep breaths and the answer will come to you while others are still panicking. You will get a reputation for being in control despite the fact that you may have done nothing more than keep your cool in the face of a crisis.

Never complain or whine in public. Although you may be reacting to real issues, responding this way in your career role will make you come across as negative and unwilling to do what needs to be done.

Identify what tasks are important and what is merely busy work. Busy work may be easier and less risky to complete but it will not accomplish important things. Find out what needs to be done in your organization and then put all your energy into doing the important things rather than the trivial things.

Develop a bias for action. Learn to act quickly and decisively. If you keep up on the current knowledge in the field, your decisions will be the right ones and you will not have to take time to analyze things.

Develop an ability to complete projects or get to the finish line regardless of the obstacles. Completing a project will give you a feeling of accomplishment. The more projects you complete, the more times you experience this feeling and the more energetic and enthusiastic you get. If you procrastinate or do not complete projects or tasks, you will feel frustrated, depressed, and disillusioned. Get the job done even if you do not do it perfectly.

Develop a habit of catching others and yourself doing things right and then acknowledge them. If you do this, you will automatically become a hero because you will help others develop a positive self-image and because they will respect and admire you for recognizing their contributions.

Read at least one professional book every two weeks. The average person reads only one professional book in their field per year (Tracy, 1986). This will give you a significant competitive edge over your fellow professionals and will allow you to fulfill your executive role and responsibilities successfully.

As a leader, your product or service is your knowledge base, skills, and access to information. Because the knowledge base is changing so quickly, professional growth and development is an ongoing process. Even if you have completed a Master's or terminal doctorate degree, you must continue your personal and professional development.

A commitment to excellence is not for the weak at heart. It

requires a significant amount of personal courage to overcome the fear of failure and rejection by others who have no desire to be excellent. These people will try to bring you down to their level. People who are not willing to pay the price to be excellent may try to sabotage and undermine your efforts in order to maintain the status quo. You need to develop enough personal courage to ward off their attempts to reject you and discredit you, and to stimulate you to question your own abilities. At times, you may feel like Christopher Columbus trying to prove that the world is round while everyone around you is trying to convince you that you are crazy because it is really flat.

The future of our health care organizations belongs to the risk-takers, and taking risks requires personal courage and a strong, positive self-image. Are you up to the challenge? Real leaders expect to experience obstacles and temporary setbacks before they get to their goals. They never view setbacks as failures or consider giving up their goals. Rather, they view each obstacle as a lesson they need to learn to get to their goal faster.

THE NURSE EXECUTIVE'S RESPONSIBILITY FOR THE IMAGE OF NURSING

Leah Curtin (1985), in a salient editorial entitled "Griping and Grousing About Nursing," stated that the negativism and defeatism in nursing was a greater problem for the profession than sexism or the issue of entry to practice. This negativity is exhibited in many studies that report that nurses view themselves as powerless. Curtin noted that even Abigail Van Buren ("Dear Abby") observed that nurses were the most frustrated and angry group of people she had ever encountered. To put things in perspective, Curtin pointed out two facts: first, on the average, nurses make more money than most working adults; second, nurses as a group have less education than any other group of professionals.

Anyone who wants success has to work long and hard hours, usually fifty to sixty hours per week. Over and above ensuring that appropriate nursing staff, models of care, and care delivery systems are in place to provide quality patient care outcomes, nurse executives have the responsibility to intervene in order to enhance the professional self-image of all the nurses in the organization.

These interventions can take many different forms. For example, the nurse executive should ensure that each nursing unit has a professional leader who role models professional responsibility, accountability, and behavior all of the time. If this is not the case, the nurse executive has the responsibility to change the leader as soon as legally feasible and possible.

The nurse executive must always role model the values of the organization and the profession. When nurse managers appear frustrated, disenchanted, and negative, the nurse executive must look into the mirror and take responsibility for that behavior. Followers always role model the behaviors and performance of their leaders.

The nurse executive must provide individual career counseling and professional feedback for individual nurses and for the whole nursing staff. All excellent nurse executives spend a significant portion of their time in career counseling activities with their staffs.

Nurse executives need to provide formal professional self-image and goal-setting training programs for their staff to give them insight into the relationship between professional self-image, behavior, and performance.

Nurse executives should share professional journal articles, books, and tapes with their nursing staff to assist them in actualizing successful professional careers.

SUMMARY

The responsibility for enhancing the professional image of nursing rests solely on the shoulders of the leaders in the profession. Nursing leaders must stop blaming the government, physicians, the public, and the educational system for the poor image of nursing.

Nurse executives have the responsibility and accountability to develop their own positive professional self-image and then to implement interventions in their organizations to teach their nurses how to enhance their own self-images as competent, contributing professionals.

7

Developing Political Skills to Enhance the Influence of Nursing

This chapter outlines the impact that enhancing the professional self-images of individual nurses can have on the profession and presents specific political skills that nurses need to develop so that the profession can take a leadership role in the health care industry.

THE IMPACT OF ENHANCED PROFESSIONAL SELF-IMAGE ON THE PROFESSION

This book is based on the assumption that the public image of the profession of nursing cannot improve until the self-image of individual nurses is enhanced. The preceding chapters focused on how self-image influences the quality of one's performance and contributions and presented concrete plans of action that nurses functioning in different roles may take to enhance their professional self-images.

The challenge to enhance the image of individual nurses and the profession will not be accomplished overnight. However, when individual nurses make progress, the image of the profession will begin to reap the rewards of their increased respect, influence, and prestige. The enhanced status of women in society will promote this process. Nurse leaders who role model these expectations will be a second

KEY CHAPTER CONCEPTS

Key Concept #1

The image of the nursing profession is directly related to the professional self-image of individual nurses.

Key Concept #2

Your ability to be successful in the political process is directly related to your self-image.

strong force that will add momentum to the process. Progress will not be fast enough or complete enough for many, but any progress toward the goal of an enhanced image will make a significant contribution to the profession and the health care industry.

EXCHANGE DISCIPLINES

Your interpersonal communications and relationships are only as good as your perception of and relationship with yourself. If you do not relate well to yourself, you cannot relate well to others. If you cannot communicate openly and honestly with yourself on controversial issues, you will be unable to communicate well with others on controversial issues.

If you have difficulty communicating and relating with others, you will not be successful in participating in routine exchange disciplines or processes. Exchange disciplines are defined as situations in which two or more people agree to exchange information, products, or services for mutual benefit. Exchange disciplines include negotiating, sales, marriage, friendship, employment relationships, and politics.

Each of the exchange disciplines relies on good communication and interpersonal skills to be effective. If you have a poor or negative self-image, your communication and interpersonal skills are compromised, and you will have difficulty being successful participating in the exchange disciplines. You will have difficulty successfully negotiating raises, maintaining happy and productive marriage and work relationships, and selling others on your ideas.

NETWORKING TO ENHANCE EFFECTIVENESS

After you have spent significant time and energy enhancing your professional self-image, dedicate some time and energy to networking with fellow professionals to influence your career and the profession of nursing. Networking is not a new concept; however, it is a skill that some women have not had much formal or informal guidance in.

A network is defined as a system of interconnected or cooperating individuals. Typically, female nurses have maintained narrow networks composed of members of their immediate work group or clinical specialty. People within work groups often think very similarly because of their close and daily exposure to one another. The attitude and thinking of the work group also is directly related to the attitude and thinking of its day-to-day leader.

Limiting yourself to such a narrow network limits you to the ideas, attitudes, and power base of a small group. To be truly effective, it is important to expand your networking beyond your immediate work group. In most instances, the problems and frustrations of your immediate work group are a function of the power and authority outside of the group. Therefore, you need to expand your networking efforts beyond the work group to be able to cope with major frustrations or the influence of others. You will gain a sense of control over issues that normally create frustration for you by expanding your networking influence.

Once you have enhanced your professional self-image, you will have developed the confidence and perspective to network with professionals outside your immediate work group. Without a strong sense of self as a valuable professional, however, you will not seek others out to solve problems and negotiate solutions. You will be able to relate with confidence to other professionals on potentially controversial issues only after developing a strong sense of self as a valuable, contributing professional.

As you pursue your professional goals, you will also be assisting the profession to accomplish its goal of enhancing its image. To help you to accomplish your goals, Display 7-1 provides a list of networks in the health care industry that can benefit you if you participate in them.

Display 7-1
NETWORKS IN THE HEALTH CARE INDUSTRY

Network	Benefits
Employees in other departments	Feedback on your department; job opportunities in other departments; innovative ideas to solve old problems; access to information
Nurses in other organizations	Job opportunities; clinical advancements; innovative ideas; sample programs and policies; mentor relationships; clinical validation and feedback
Professional organizations	Community standards in clinical practice; job opportunities; leadership opportunities; role models; expanded power base
Nurse managers	Mentor relationships; career opportunities; role models

(continued)

ORGANIZING FOR POLITICAL IMPACT

Politics can be defined as acquiring the monetary and the human resources that are necessary to influence the allocation of limited resources in a specific system. The system can be your department, organization, profession, industry, city, state, etc. Depending on the specific system you deal with, you need to develop specific contacts to influence the allocation of scarce resources in that system. The smaller the system, the fewer the number of contacts needed to accomplish

Display 7-1 *(continued)*
NETWORKS IN THE HEALTH CARE INDUSTRY

Network	*Benefits*
Nurse executives	Career opportunities; career advice; exchange of information and perceptions
Health care administrators	Opportunity to be heard; opportunity to receive information; opportunity to influence decision-makers
Legislative representatives	Opportunity to air views and perspectives on health care issues; opportunity to understand system; opportunity to serve on a committee
Successful businesspeople	Observe specific success traits in action; learn business strategies; mentor relationships

your goals. As a system expands in size, the number and diversity of contacts you need to influence increases significantly, as well as the level of energy and effort required to influence the system. Most people wish to influence larger systems. They usually do not do a good job in this area because they lack the time, energy, and commitment required to influence large systems.

The profession needs more nurses who are confident in their professional roles and who invest the time and energy to network with other professionals within and outside of their immediate work group to enhance the image of the profession. This political activity needs to occur in a professional atmosphere that is not accompanied by overwhelming emotion. Political action needs to be an ongoing activity in which nurses are engaged throughout their professional careers at varying levels, based on the current issues.

LOBBYING:
A PROFESSIONAL RESPONSIBILITY

Lobbying is a means of exercising group power to accomplish specific goals. A group's power can contribute to a positive image for the profession to which it belongs.

People usually need to make the transition to being internally driven and believe that they can affect their external environment and the legislative process before they get involved in lobbying. This belief is possible only when a person has assumed total responsibility for self and professional satisfaction and has developed a strong, positive professional self-image.

Effective lobbying is directly related to (1) the amount of money spent by an organization; (2) the level of sophistication of the lobbying efforts; and (3) the size, location, and socioeconomic status of the group (Bushy & Smith, 1990).

To be successful in any lobbying effort, the nursing profession must take a number of actions, including

1. Taking personal responsibility for committing the time and financial resources to support legislative issues affecting health care.
2. Acquiring the knowledge and skills required to participate in the legislative process.
3. Compromising individual beliefs to support the goals of the nursing profession on issues in order to make the voice of the profession heard.
4. Becoming a leader and role model to expand the influence of nursing and to educate future nurse leaders on their legislative responsibility.
5. Actively supporting professional nurse lobbying efforts by taking the time to make telephone calls and write letters to legislators and provide oral testimony when called upon to do so. These efforts sometimes also require running the risk of being considered controversial among and by your peers. No great things are accomplished

without taking risks. You must take risks on behalf of your career and profession, because you only get out of it what you've put in first.

6. Actively supporting professional legislative efforts through financial contributions to health care political action committees. If you never contribute on behalf of an issue or cause, you have no business complaining about why your voice is not heard or things never change.

Most nurses are unfamiliar with lobbying and the legislative process for a number of reasons. One reason is that the profession is more than 96% women, while legislative activities have historically been dominated by men (Hunter, 1984).

A second reason is that the female-dominated profession of nursing historically has been more externally than internally driven. Because of this, many nurses perceive that they are controlled by external factors and that they do not have the power to affect their external environment significantly. For years they have felt that they could not change the policies and procedures within their own departments, let alone the bureaucracy of their organizations. Therefore, they feel it would be a waste of time trying to affect the large and powerful legislative arena. This perception deters many nurses from actively participating in legislative issues unless they perceive a particular issue as a crisis issue.

A third reason for the low level of nurse involvement and presence in the legislative process is the general lack of skill in and understanding of the process. This is because nurses are not significantly exposed to the process in traditional nurse education and work place experiences. Women in general tend to avoid situations and arenas in which they possess little expertise because they have been socialized to avoid risk and to seek secure situations. Traditional gender socialization has also taught them that men take care of legislative issues. Historically, there have been few female role models to emulate in the legislative arena. As a result, many women perceive that this activity is out of their domain. This is similar to the commonly held perception that women could not become physicians. This belief was prevalent until about ten years ago. Today, 40% to 50% of all medical school enrollees are women, a fact which has changed this commonly held perception. As more and more women enter the legislative arena, the common perception that this is not a woman's arena will also change.

A fourth reason nurses have not been a prominent force in the legislative arena is that they have not been able to agree on many things as a group. There are a number of nurse activist projects underway, but fragmentation has occurred because of the many different nursing organizations that claim to speak for the profession, including the American Nurses Association, the American Organization of Nurse Executives, the American Association of Operating Room Nurses, the American Association of Critical Care Nurses, and the National League for Nursing. This fragmentation has diluted the influence of the profession as a whole because these groups sometimes hold conflicting views on basic issues.

After large numbers of individual nurses take the actions outlined in this book to enhance their own professional self-image and maximize their professional performance and contributions, I believe that the image of the profession can be enhanced. As the image of the profession is enhanced, nurses will be more able to compromise and negotiate to establish common ground and goals to unite them on core issues.

SUMMARY

The image of the profession can be enhanced when a significant number of nurses have enhanced their individual professional self-images and have networked with colleagues.

Traditionally, many nurses have had poor professional self-images and have not sought out contacts outside their immediate work groups because of their feelings of inferiority. They also have not routinely met with fellow professionals to communicate on a proactive and supportive note.

As individual nurses enhance their professional self-images, the collective image of the profession will reflect that change. Professions are made up of individual people, and outsiders perceive the profession through these people. As a nurse, you have a responsibility to yourself and the profession to be the best professional you can be.

Bibliography

Anderson, M. L. (1983). *Thinking about women: Sociological and feminist perspectives*. New York: MacMillan.

Bachtold, L. M. (1976). Personality characteristics of women of achievement. *Psychology of Women Quarterly, 1*, 70.

Bandura, A. (1977). *Social learning theory*. Englewood Cliffs, NJ: Prentice-Hall.

Bardwick, J. M. (1971). *Psychology of women*. New York: Harper & Row.

Bardwick, J. M., & Douvan, E. (1971). Ambivalence: The socialization of women. In Vivian Gornick & Barbara K. Moran (Eds.), *Woman in a sexist society*. New York: Basic Books.

Baruch, G. K. (1976). Girls who perceive themselves as competent: Some antecedents and correlates. *Psychology of Women Quarterly, 1*, 38.

Beattie, M. (1987). *Co-dependent no more*. Center City, MN: Hazelden Foundation.

Bedeian, A., & Touliatos, J. (1978). Work-related motives and self-esteem in American women. *Journal of Psychology, 99*, 63.

Bem, S. L. (1974). The measurement of psychological androgyny. *Journal of Consulting and Clinical Psychology, 42*, 155–162.

Bennis, W., & Nanus, B. (1985). *Leaders*. New York: Harper & Row.

Benziger, K. (1985, May/June). The powerful woman. *Hospital Forum*, pp. 15–20.

Brockner, J. (1988). The effects of work layoffs on supervisors: Research, theory, and practice. In B. M. Staw & L. L. Cummings (Eds.), *Research in organizational behavior* (Vol. 10, pp. 213–255). Greenwich, CT: JAI Press.

Brockner, J., Derr, W. R., & Laing, W. N. (1987). Self-esteem and reactions to negative feedback: Towards greater generalizability. *Journal of Research in Personality, 21*: 318–333.

Brockner, J., & Elkind, M. (1985). Self-esteem and reactance: Further evidence of attitudinal and motivational consequences. *Journal of Experimental Social Psychology, 21*, 346–361.

Brockner, J., & Rubin, J. Z. (1985). *Entrapment in escalating conflicts: A social psychological analysis*. New York: Springer-Verlag.

Broome, J. H. (1963). *Rousseau: A study of his thought*. London: Edward Arnold.

Broverman, I. K., Broverman, D. M., Clarkson, F. E., Rosenkrantz, P. S., & Vogel, S. R. (1970). Sex role stereotypes and clinical judgements of mental health. *Journal of Counseling and Clinical Psychology, 34*, 1–7.

Brown, D. G. (1956). Sex role preference in young children. *Psychological Monographs, 70*(14).

Bushy, A., & Smith, T. O. (1990, April). Lobbying: The how's and wherefores. *Nursing Management*, pp. 39–45.

Byrne, S. K. (1982). Accepting the "red." In J. Muff (Ed.), *Socialization, sexism, and stereotyping*. Prospect Heights, IL: Waveland Press.

CAHHS (1989). *California Association of Hospital and Healthcare Systems 1989* report.

Carlzon, J. (1987). *Moments of truth*. Cambridge, MA: Ballinger.

Carroll, S. J., & Tosi, H. L. (1970). Goal characteristics and personality factors in a management-by-objective program. *Administrative Science Quarterly, 15*, 295–305.

Chernin, K. (1981). *The obsession*. New York: Harper & Row.

Chesler, P. (1972). *Women and madness*. New York: Avon Books.

Chodorow, N. (1974). Family structure and feminine personality. In M. Z. Rosaldo & L. Lamphere (Eds.), *Woman, culture, and society*. Stanford, CA: Stanford University Press.

Chodorow, N. (1978). *The reproduction of mothering*. Berkeley: University of California Press.

Cialdini, R. B., & Richardson, K. D. (1980). Two indirect tactics of impression management: Basking and blasting. *Journal of Personality and Social Psychology, 39*, 406–415.

Clark, M. D. (1986). The historical basis for nursing's troubled self-image. *Journal of the American Association of Occupational Health Nursing, 34*(4), 169–170.

Coopersmith, S. (1967). *The antecedents of self-esteem*. San Francisco: W. H. Freeman.

Cummings, L. D. (1977). Value stretching in definitions of career among college women: Horatio Alger as a feminist model. *Social Problems, 25*(1), 65.

Curtin, L. (1985). Griping and grousing about nursing [editorial]. *Nursing Management*, *16*(8), 7–8.

Dean, P. G. (1988). Toward androgyny. In J. Muff (Ed.), *Socialization, sexism, and stereotyping*. Prospect Heights, IL: Waveland Press.

Deaux, K., White, L., & Farris, E. (1975). Skill versus luck: Field and laboratory studies of male and female preferences. *Journal of Personality and Social Psychology*, *32*, 629–636.

Deutsch, H. (1944). *The psychology of women* (Vol. 2). New York: Grune & Stratton.

Dowling, C. (1982). *The cinderella complex*. New York: Pocket Books.

Dowling, C. (1984). *Perfect women*. New York: Pocket Books.

Dweck, C. S. (1975). The role of expectations and attributions in the alienation of learned helplessness. *Journal of Personality and Social Psychology*, *31*, 674–685.

Erikson, E. H. (1980). *Identity and the life cycle*. New York & London: W. W. Norton.

Flannelly, L., & Flannelly, K. (1984). The masculine and feminine in nursing. *Nursing Forum*, *21*(4), 162–165.

Friedan, B. (1974). *The feminine mystique*. New York: W. W. Norton.

Garfield, C. (1986). *Peak performers*. New York: Avon Books.

Gilligan, C. (1982). *In a different voice: Psychological theory and women's development*. Cambridge, MA & London: Harvard University Press.

Greene, C. N., & Organ, D. W. (1973). An evaluation of causal models linking the perceived role with job satisfaction. *Administrative Science Quarterly*, *18*, 95–103.

Hardy, M. E. (1978). Role stress and role strain. In M. E. Hardy & M. E. Conway (Eds.), *Role theory*. New York: Appleton-Century-Crofts.

Hartley, R. E. (1959). Sex-role pressures and socialization of the male child. *Psychological Reports*, *5*, 457.

Heilbrun, A. B., Jr. (1958). Sex role, instrumental-expressive behavior and psychopathology in females. *Journal of Abnormal Psychology*, *73*(2), 131.

Helgesen, S. (1990). *The female advantage: Women's ways of leadership*. New York: Doubleday.

Hennig, M. (1974). Family dynamics and the successful woman executive. In R. Knudsin (Ed.), *Women and success*. New York: William Morrow.

Henry, B., & LeClair, H. (1987). Language, leadership and power. *Journal of Nursing Administration*, *17* (1), 19–25.

Hoffman, L. W. (1972). Early childhood experiences and woman's achievement motives. *Journal of Social Issues*, *28*, 129.

Horner, M. S. (1972). Toward an understanding of achievement related conflicts in women. *Journal of Social Issues*, *28*, 157–175.

Horner, M. S., & Walsh, M. P. (1974). Psychological barriers to success in women. In R. Knudsin, *Women and success*. New York: William Morrow.

Hunter, P. (1984). Regulation and nursing in California. *Nursing Administration Quarterly, 8*(4), 61–69.

Journard, S. M. (1974). Some lethal aspects of the male role. In J. Pleckland & J. Sawyer (Eds.), *Men and masculinity*. Englewood Cliffs, NJ: Spectrum Books.

Kagan, J., & Moss, H. A. (1962). *Birth to maturity: A study of psychological development*. New York: John Wiley.

Kalisch, S. J., & Kalisch, P. A. (1982). The nurse as a sex object in motion pictures, 1930 to 1980. *Research Nurse Health, 5*(3), 147–154.

Kanter, R. M. (1977). *Men and women of the corporation*. New York: Basic Books.

Kanter, R. M. (1989). *When giants learn to dance*. New York: Simon & Schuster.

Kluckholn, C. (1962). *Culture and behavior*. New York: Free Press.

Kobasa, S. C. (1979). Stressful life events, personality, and health: An inquiry into hardiness. *Journal of Personality and Social Psychology, 37*(1), 1–11.

Kohn, M. I., & Schooler, C. (1983). *Work and personality: An inquiry into the impact of social stratification*. Norwood, NJ: Ablex.

Korman, A. K. (1966). Self-esteem variable in vocational choice. *Journal of Applied Psychology, 50*, 479–486.

Korman, A. K. (1970). Toward a hypothesis of work behavior. *Journal of Applied Psychology, 54*, 31–41.

Kramer, M. (1987). Magnet hospitals. *Nursing Management, 18*(9 & 10).

Ladner, J. (1971). *Tomorrow's tomorrow*. Garden City, NY: Doubleday-Anchor.

Lever, J. (1976). Sex differences in the games children play. *Social Problems, 23*, 478–487.

Maccoby, E. E., & Jacklin, C. N. (1974). *The psychology of sex differences* (Vol. 1). Stanford, CA: Stanford University Press.

Mahler, M. S. (1979). *Selected papers of Margaret S. Mahler, M.D.: Vol. 2: Separation individuation*. New York: Jason Aaronsen.

Maltz, M. (1975). *Psychocybernetics*. New York: Warner Books.

Mead, G. H. (1934). *Mind, self, and society*. Chicago: University of Chicago Press.

Morrison, R. F. (1977). Career adaptability: The effective adaptation of managers to changing role demands. *Journal of Applied Psychology, 62*, 549–558.

Mossholder, K. W., Bedian, A. G., & Armenakis, A. A. (1981). Role perceptions, satisfaction, and performance: Moderating effects of self-esteem and organizational level. *Organizational Behavior and Human Performance, 28*, 224–234.

Muff, J. (1982). *Socialization, sexism, and stereotyping: Women's issues in nursing*. Prospect Heights, IL: Waveland Press.

Norwood, R. (1985). *Women who love too much*. Los Angeles: Jeremy P. Tarcher.

Olsen, E. (1988, December). Beyond positive thinking. *Success*, pp. 31–32.

Peters, T. (1987). *Thriving on chaos*. New York: Alfred A. Knopf.

Pierce. J. V. (1961). *Sex differences in achievement motivation of able high school students* (Cooperative research project No. 1097). Chicago: University of Chicago.

Pondy, L. J. (1978). Leadership is a language game. In M. W. McCall & M. M. Lombardo (Eds.), *Leadership, where else can we go?* (pp. 94–95). Durham, NC: Duke University Press.

Puetz, B. E. (1983). *Networking for nurses*. Rockville, MD: Aspen Systems Corporation.

Rabban, M. L. (1950). Sex role identification in young children in two diverse social groups. *Genetic Psychological Monographs, 42*, 81.

Rheingold, H. L., & Cook, K. V. (1975). The contents of boys' and girls' rooms as an index of parents' behavior. *Child Development, 46*, 459–463.

Roberts, S. J. (1983). Oppressed group behavior: Implications for nursing. *Advances in Nursing Science*, (4) 21–30.

Rodgers, J. A. (1981, August). Toward professional adulthood. *Nursing Outlook*, pp. 478–481.

Rogers, C. R. (1961). *On becoming a person*. Boston: Houghton-Mifflin.

Rosenberg, M. (1979). *Conceiving the self*. New York: Basic Books.

Rosenthal, R., & Jacobson, L. (1968). *Pygmalion in the classroom: Teacher expectation and pupils' intellectual development*. New York: Holt, Rinehart, & Winston.

Rubin, L. (1976). *Worlds of pain: Life in the working class family*. New York: Basic Books.

Sanford, L. T., & Donovan, M. E. (1984). *Women and self-esteem*. Baltimore: Penguin Books.

Scalzi, C. C. (1988). Role stress and coping strategies of nurse executives. *Journal of Nursing Administration, 18*(3), 34–37.

Schwartz, J. P. (1986, March). Are women better managers? *Success*, 19–20.

Siegel, B. (1989). *Peace, love, and healing*. New York: Harper & Row.

Singer, J. (1976). *Androgyny, the opposites within*. Boston: Sigo Press.

Spence, J., Helmreich, R., & Stapp, J. (1975). Ratings of self and peers on sex role attributes and their relation to self esteem and concepts of masculinity and femininity. *Journal of Personality and Social Psychology, 31*, 29.

Spence J. T., & Helmreich, R. (1978). *Masculinity and femininity: Their psychological dimensions, correlations, and antecedents*. Austin, TX: University of Texas Press.

Strasen, L. L. (1987). *Key business skills for nurse managers*. Philadelphia: J. B. Lippincott.

Symonds, A. (1976, April). Neurotic dependency in successful women. *Journal of the American Academy of Psychoanalysis*, pp. 95–103.

Tavris, C., & Offir, C. (1977). *The longest war*. New York: Harcourt Brace Jovanovich.

Tharenou, R. (1979). Employee self-esteem: A review of the literature. *Journal of Vocational Behavior, 15*, 316–346.

Tolson, A. (1977). *The limits of masculinity*. New York: Harper.

Tracy, B. (1986). *The psychology of achievement*. Chicago, IL: Nightengale Conant.

Vaillant, G. E. (1979). Natural history of male psychologic health: Effects of mental health on physical health. *New England Journal of Medicine, 301*(23).

Witt & Associates (1987). *Profile of a nurse executive*. Chicago, IL: Author.

Index